THE NEW ULTIMATE STROKE DIET COOKBOOK FOR BEGINNERS

100+ Nutritional Recipes, Healthy Meal Plan and Essential Guide for Stroke Recovery

PATRICK BRYANT

Table of Contents

INTRODUCTION

Stroke is one of the most leading reasons of disabilities and death all over the world. The incidence of stroke in high income countries descended from 163-94 cases per 100,000 person years, between 1970 and 2008. This decrease coincided with increased public awareness of the dangers to health, which is posed by elevated blood pressure, high blood cholesterol, cigarette smoking, and reduced prevalence of these risk-factors in the population. The estimation of the World health organization that between 1990 and 2020, the stroke mortality will enhance by 78% in woman and 106% in man. Nutrition plays much more important role in the stroke prevention than it is appreciated by most physicians and nutritionists. The aim of the present paper is to explain the evidences, which link nutrition to the stroke risk.

Diet is an important part of recovery following a stroke. It may involve making changes to help prevent further strokes, as well as adjustments that accommodate any symptoms a person has, such as difficulty swallowing.

Diet for stroke prevention typically involves eating lots of fruits and vegetables, lean protein, whole grains, and foods low in added salt. Some people recovering from a stroke may also have other health conditions that require dietary changes, such as diabetes or high blood pressure. As these conditions may have contributed to the stroke, it is important to also address them.

Understanding Stroke Recovery and Nutrition

Understanding stroke recovery involves recognizing the importance of nutrition in the healing process. After a stroke, the body requires nutrients to repair damaged tissues, support brain function, and prevent complications. Here are key considerations for stroke recovery and nutrition:

• Focus on Nutrient-Dense Foods: Emphasize a diet rich in fruits, vegetables, whole grains, lean proteins, and healthy fats. These foods provide essential nutrients, antioxidants, and fiber to support overall health and aid in recovery.

• Manage Blood Pressure and Cholesterol: Opt for low-sodium foods to help control blood pressure and reduce the risk of another stroke. Choose heart-healthy fats like those found in nuts, seeds, avocados, and olive oil to improve cholesterol levels.

• Maintain a Healthy Weight: Balance calorie intake with physical activity to achieve and maintain a healthy weight. Excess weight can increase the risk of complications and hinder recovery after a stroke.

• Stay Hydrated: Drink plenty of water throughout the day to stay hydrated, which is essential for overall health and optimal recovery.

• Consider Dysphagia Management: If swallowing difficulties (dysphagia) are present after a stroke, work with a healthcare professional or speech therapist to modify food textures and ensure safe swallowing.

• Monitor Blood Sugar Levels: For individuals with diabetes or those at risk of developing diabetes, monitor blood sugar levels closely and choose foods with a low glycemic index to help control blood sugar.

• Limit Alcohol and Caffeine: Reduce consumption of alcohol and caffeinated beverages, as they can interfere with medications and exacerbate certain stroke-related symptoms.

• Seek Guidance from Healthcare Professionals: Consult with a registered dietitian or nutritionist who specializes in stroke recovery to develop a personalized meal plan tailored to individual needs and goals.

By prioritizing nutrient-dense foods, managing key health indicators like blood pressure and cholesterol, and seeking guidance from healthcare professionals, individuals can support their recovery and enhance overall well-being after a stroke.

Overview of Stroke and Its Effects

A stroke occurs when blood flow to part of the brain is interrupted, leading to damage of brain cells due to lack of oxygen and nutrients. There are two main types of stroke:

• Ischemic Stroke: This occurs when a blood vessel supplying blood to the brain is blocked by a blood clot or plaque buildup. Ischemic strokes account for the majority of stroke cases.

• Hemorrhagic Stroke: This occurs when a blood vessel in the brain ruptures and causes bleeding into or around the brain. Hemorrhagic strokes are less common but often more severe.

The effects of a stroke can vary widely depending on factors such as the location and severity of the brain damage, as well as how quickly medical treatment is received. Common effects of stroke may include:

• Weakness or Paralysis: This often affects one side of the body and can range from mild weakness to complete paralysis.

• Speech and Language Difficulties: Aphasia, difficulty speaking or understanding language, and dysarthria, difficulty controlling the muscles used in speech, are common after a stroke.

• Cognitive Impairments: Stroke survivors may experience difficulties with memory, attention, problem-solving, and other cognitive functions.

• Vision Problems: Visual disturbances or loss of vision in one or both eyes can occur after a stroke.

• Emotional and Behavioral Changes: Depression, anxiety, mood swings, and changes in personality are common psychological effects of stroke.

• Physical and Sensory Changes: Other effects may include pain, numbness, tingling, or changes in sensation in affected areas of the body.

Stroke rehabilitation aims to help individuals regain as much function and independence as possible through various therapies and interventions, including physical therapy, occupational therapy, speech therapy, and psychological support. Early recognition of stroke symptoms and prompt medical treatment are crucial for improving outcomes and minimizing long-term effects.

The Role of Nutrition in Stroke Recovery

Nutrition plays a crucial role in stroke recovery, as it supports overall health, aids in healing, and can help prevent complications. Here's how nutrition contributes to stroke recovery:

• Supports Brain Health: Nutrient-rich foods provide essential vitamins, minerals, and antioxidants that support brain function and repair damaged tissue. Foods high in omega-3 fatty acids, such as fish, nuts, and seeds, are particularly beneficial for brain health.

• Manages Blood Pressure and Cholesterol: A diet low in sodium and saturated fats can help manage blood pressure and cholesterol levels, reducing the risk of further cardiovascular complications, including recurrent strokes.

• Promotes Heart Health: Heart-healthy foods, such as fruits, vegetables, whole grains, and lean proteins, can help maintain cardiovascular health, which is essential for stroke recovery and prevention.

• Aids in Weight Management: A balanced diet rich in fiber and protein can help individuals achieve and maintain a healthy weight, reducing the risk of obesity-related complications and improving overall well-being.

• Addresses Swallowing Difficulties: For individuals with swallowing difficulties (dysphagia) following a stroke, modifying food textures and ensuring adequate hydration are essential for safe and effective nutrition.

• Controls Blood Sugar Levels: For individuals with diabetes or those at risk of developing diabetes, monitoring blood sugar levels and choosing foods with a low glycemic index can help control blood sugar and prevent complications.

• Supports Energy Levels and Recovery: Eating regular, balanced meals and staying hydrated can help maintain energy levels and support the body's healing processes during stroke recovery.

• Reduces Inflammation: Anti-inflammatory foods, such as fruits, vegetables, and omega-3 fatty acids, can help reduce inflammation in the body, which may aid in stroke recovery and reduce the risk of future cardiovascular events.

Overall, a well-balanced diet that prioritizes nutrient-dense foods is essential for stroke recovery. Working with a registered dietitian or nutritionist can help individuals develop a personalized meal plan tailored to their specific needs and goals during the recovery process.

How This Cookbook Can Help You

This cookbook can be a valuable resource for individuals seeking to improve their health and well-being through nutritious and delicious meals. Here's how it can help you:

• Inspiring Recipes: The cookbook provides a diverse range of recipes, from quick and easy meals to more elaborate dishes, to inspire creativity and enjoyment in the kitchen.

• Nutritional Guidance: Each recipe is crafted with nutritional balance in mind, providing essential nutrients while emphasizing whole foods and healthy ingredients.

• Health Focus: Whether you're looking to manage a specific health condition, lose weight, or simply adopt a healthier lifestyle, the cookbook offers recipes tailored to various dietary needs and goals.

• Meal Planning Support: With a variety of breakfast, lunch, dinner, and snack options, the cookbook can assist with meal planning, helping you stay organized and prepared throughout the week.

• Educational Content: Alongside recipes, the cookbook may include educational content on nutrition, cooking techniques, ingredient substitutions, and more, empowering you to make informed choices about your diet and health.

• Variety and Flexibility: Whether you follow a specific dietary pattern like vegan, gluten-free, or paleo, or simply enjoy exploring new flavors and cuisines, the cookbook offers a wide array of options to suit your taste preferences and dietary restrictions.

• Family-Friendly Options: With recipes designed to appeal to individuals of all ages, the cookbook can help you create wholesome and satisfying meals that the whole family will enjoy.

• Cooking Confidence: By providing clear instructions, helpful tips, and beautiful photography, the cookbook can boost your confidence in the kitchen, making cooking an enjoyable and rewarding experience.

Overall, this cookbook serves as a valuable tool for anyone looking to enhance their culinary skills, expand their recipe repertoire, and prioritize their health and well-being through nourishing and flavorful meals.

The Diet for stroke prevention

One of the main aims of diets for people who have had a stroke is helping prevent future strokes. The Mediterranean diet is a common approach to this. It involves focusing on fresh produce, lean protein, and healthy fats such as olive oil.

The American Heart Association (AHA) recommends eating:

• a variety of fruits and vegetables, ideally fresh, frozen, or canned

• whole grains, such as brown rice, oats, quinoa, and barley

• legumes, such as beans, peas, and lentils

• lean proteins, such as chicken or tofu

• oily fish, such as salmon, sardines, or herring

• unsaturated fats, such as olive oil or avocado oil

• low fat dairy products, such as yogurt or skim milk

• nuts and seeds

Be mindful that some types of fish contain more mercury than others. Smaller fish, such as sardines, contain beneficial nutrients without harmful levels of mercury. A person may wish to aim to eat these twice a week.

Some foods to reduce or avoid include:

• highly processed baked goods, such as white bread, cakes, and pastries

• foods high in saturated fats, such as red meat and full-fat dairy

• foods that contain added sugars, such as sucrose, high fructose corn syrup, brown sugar, or molasses

• foods high in added salt

Diet for swallowing difficulties

Some people experience difficulty swallowing, or dysphagia, after a stroke.

The AHA suggests ways of modifying recipes to accommodate the needs of adults who have had a stroke. The suggestions align with the International Dysphagia Diet Standardization Initiative, which describes different food consistencies people can use based on how severe the symptoms are. They include the following:

• Level 4 modifications involve pureeing food so that chewing is not necessary.

• Level 5 foods are minced and moist, so they do not require biting.

• Level 6 foods are soft and bite-sized so that a person can safely chew and swallow the food.

• Level 7 includes regular foods that a person can eat as they typically would.

Foods that people can easily change into one of the above consistencies include:

• scrambled eggs

• baked fish, such as salmon

• minced meat, such as chicken or turkey

• root vegetables, such as carrots

• potatoes

• avocados

• oatmeal

• yogurt

• banana

A person's medical team can also help with identifying what modifications are appropriate.

Other tips that may help with preparing softer foods include:

• cooking vegetables in water so they soften, rather than roasting or frying them

• sieving or straining foods to remove pips, seeds, husks, or skins

• cooking meat until it is very tender

Diet for helping prevent weight loss

Losing weight is a common side effect of a stroke, and it can have a negative effect on stroke outcomes. Diet is an important aspect of managing this, and it can help a person maintain or gain weight.

Nutrient-dense foods that contain a high number of calories in each portion can help prevent weight loss. Many of these are also adaptable for people with dysphagia. They include:

• avocado

• banana

• soft cheeses

• yogurt

A person may also wish to try nut or seed butters. However, when trying these, it is important to ensure the consistency is runny enough to swallow them easily, as some nut butters can be very thick.

Another option is high calorie smoothies or shakes. People may be able to buy formulas that are suitable for after a stroke, or it is possible to make them at home. Some ingredients that may work for this include:

• protein powders, such as whey, pea, or soy protein

• nut powders or butters

• fruits

• pasteurized egg whites

• natural sweeteners, such as dates or honey

• a liquid, such as water, milk, or plant milks

People may also be able to add extra calories to meals by:

• adding extra oil, such as olive oil

• using full-fat dairy products instead of ones that are low fat, if a doctor says doing so is safe

• trying smaller, more frequent meals instead of a few large meals

Diet for stroke patients with high blood pressure

High blood pressure is the most common stroke risk factor. Diet can help to manage it. Many of the dietary changes that can help reduce future strokes can also help with blood pressure.

It is especially important for people with high blood pressure to monitor their sodium intake. Sodium is in salt. Humans need salt to survive, though too much can be harmful.

People can use more spices and less salt to add flavor to foods. Foods that can be high in salt include:

• processed meats, such as bacon

• salty snacks, such as potato chips

• canned soups

• convenience foods, such as frozen dinners, pizzas, or spice mixes

• preserved foods, such as olives in brine

In a 2021 study, using high amounts of herbs and spices in food lowered blood pressure. The study involved 24 different herbs and spices, including:

• black pepper

• garlic

• basil

• thyme

• turmeric

• cinnamon

• chili powder

Other aspects of diet and lifestyle, such as drinking alcohol and smoking, can also affect blood pressure.

Diet for stroke patients with diabetes

Diabetes is another risk factor for a stroke, so if a person has both conditions, they will also need to consider how food will affect their blood sugar level.

It may be especially important for people in this group to limit foods that contain added sugar, such as:

• Candy and chocolate

• Ice cream

• Sweetened yogurts

• Baked goods

• Drinks with added sugar, such as soda, juices, sports drinks, or energy drinks

Some people may also need to count the overall number of carbohydrates they eat each day. This can help with managing blood sugar and determining how much insulin to use.

People can discuss managing several medical conditions through their diet with a registered dietitian. Medicare covers this for people with diabetes.

When to seek help

If it is difficult for a person recovering from a stroke to chew, swallow, or consume enough calories, they should speak with a doctor as soon as they can. A doctor may be able to offer additional help or refer them to a dietitian for further support.

People can also speak with a doctor or dietitian if they would like additional help reducing their stroke risk or managing chronic conditions through their diet.

If a person is having difficulty shopping for or preparing food, an occupational therapist may be able to help them carry out day-to-day activities with more ease. This could involve making adjustments around the house to make movement easier and using large utensils that are easier to grip, among many other potential changes.

Some resources that may help include:

• the American Stroke Association's Simply Goodonline cookbook, which is also available in Spanish

• stroke support groups, which people can find locally using this tool

• the Stroke Family Warmline, which provides support for caregivers and family members

Rehabilitation for stroke: What to know

When someone has a stroke, they should begin rehabilitation as soon as possible. Not only does it help improve the chances of making a full recovery, but it may help reduce the risk of future strokes. Prompt rehabilitation also eases the transition from hospital to home.

Stroke rehabilitation is a team effort. It involves the person who had the stroke, their family and friends, and various healthcare professionals.

The person may require support from physical and occupational therapists, speech-language therapists, neurologists, specialist nurses, and physiatrists (physical medicine and rehabilitation physicians). Together, they will develop a rehabilitation plan that meets the person's unique needs.

What is stroke rehabilitation?

Stroke rehabilitation is therapy that helps people recover from the aftereffects of a stroke.

A stroke occurs when the blood supply to part of the brain is cut off. It can occur when a blood vessel becomes blocked or bursts. When this happens, brain cells are starved of oxygen and begin to die. A stroke is a medical emergency, and prompt treatment is essential. If treatment does not occur to restore the blood supply, damage to the brain can be permanent.

The type of rehabilitation someone requires depends on the severity of the stroke and the affected areas of the brain. In general, however, the aim of rehabilitation is to help the person relearn skills that may have been lost, learn compensatory techniques where relevant, and make any necessary lifestyle changes.

What disabilities can a stroke cause?

Strokes can cause a range of disabilities, depending on the area of the brain affected. Some common problems include:
• Pain
• Difficulty reading and writing
• Memory problems
• Mood swings and emotional changes
• Paralysis or hemiparesis, which is weakness on one side of the body
• Trouble speaking or understanding language

What does stroke rehabilitation involve?

The rehabilitation process aims to help an individual regain as much function and independence as possible.

It involves a team of healthcare professionals, including:

• Doctors

• Nurses

• Therapists

• Counselors

The team develops a customized treatment plan based on the person's individual needs.

The plan may include:

• Physical therapy to help the person relearn simple motor activities, such as walking, sitting, and lying down

• Occupational therapy to help with everyday activities through exercise and training

• Speech-language therapy to help relearn language and speaking skills

• Cognitive rehabilitation to help with thinking and memory problems

• Counseling to help the person and their family cope with the emotional impact of a stroke

• Medications to help with a range of symptoms that occur as a result of a stroke

Physical activities

Most people who have had a stroke need physical activities to help them relearn movement skills and coordination they might have lost.

If the stroke affected their upper extremities more than the lower extremities, the person may require occupational therapy to help with fine motor skills. They may require physical therapy to help with gross motor skills.

For most stroke survivors, rehabilitation focuses on physical therapy.

The therapist starts by helping the person perform safe exercises, such as range-of-motion exercises and stretching.

As the person gets stronger, they progress to more challenging activities, such as walking and climbing stairs.

The therapist may help the person safely use tools such as:

• canes

• walkers

• wheelchairs

They may also use electrical stimulation and massage to help reduce pain and improve muscle function.

Cognitive rehabilitation

A person who has had a stroke may experience cognitive impairment, such as forgetfulness, disorientation, and confusion. These can negatively impact their quality of life. Following a stroke, people may experience emotional distress, such as mood swings, anxiety, and depression. Cognitive rehabilitation helps the person identify and compensate for cognitive deficits. The therapist may teach the person strategies to help with:

• memory

• attention

• problem-solving

• concentration

• daily functions, such as handling finances or medications

• processing the impact the stroke has had on their life

Technology-assisted therapy

Technology-assisted activities may include:

• computer programs

• virtual reality

• robotic devices

These activities can help the person practice new skills and improve their function.

For example, computer programs can help a person with memory problems learn how to organize information. Virtual reality can help people practice grocery shopping or cooking tasks. They may use robotic devices to help regain movement in their arms or legs.

Newer therapies

Researchers are looking into several newer therapies for their potential in stroke recovery, including:

• Constraint-induced movement therapy: This involves restraining the use of the unaffected arm or leg while working the affected limb. The aim is to help the person relearn how to use the affected limb.

• Functional electrical stimulation: This therapy uses electrical stimulationto help the person regain movement in their limbs.

• Transcranial magnetic stimulation: This therapy uses magnetic fieldsto stimulate nerve cells in the brain and improve function.

Using these alongside physical therapies or other therapy types may be beneficial.

Who is involved in the rehabilitation plan?

A team of professionals will help people during their recovery program and may comprise the following:

• Physical therapist: Helps a person regain strength, range of motion, coordination, and balance.

• Neurologist: Specializes in stroke and other conditions affecting the brain and spinal cord.

• Rehabilitation nurse: Helps a person manage any health problems and adjust to life after a stroke.

• Occupational therapist: Provides strategies that help someone manage personal care or daily activities such as cooking and eating.

• Speech-language pathologist: Helps a person with speech and language difficulties, problems reading and writing, and eating and swallowing issues.

• Dietician: Provides information about healthy eating and special dietary needs.

• Social worker: Assists people with rehabilitation programs, living arrangements, insurance, and support at home.

• Neuropsychologist: Treats issues with changes in thinking, memory, and behavior.

• Physiatrist: Assists with physical medicine and rehabilitation.

Where does rehabilitation take place?

Stroke rehabilitation can take place in various settings, including:

• inpatient rehabilitation centers

• outpatient rehabilitation centers

• specialty stroke units

• nursing homes

• assisted living facilities

• at home, through home health agencies

A person may receive therapy in more than one setting. For example, they may start with inpatient rehabilitation in the hospital and then continue with outpatient therapy at home.

How can people prevent another stroke from occurring?

If a person has a stroke, they are at increased risk of having another stroke. It is important to address the causes of the stroke to reduce this risk. Causes include:

• heart disease

• high blood pressure

• atrial fibrillation

• high cholesterol

• diabetes

A doctor may prescribe medications to help these conditions. They may also recommend dietary changes, increased physical activity, and other lifestyle changes.

Frequently asked questions

Below are some of the most frequently asked questions and answers about rehabilitation from stroke.

What factors might affect the outcome of rehabilitation?

The chances of a successful recovery following a stroke depend on many factors, including:
- The severity of the stroke
- The person's age and overall health
- How soon treatment starts
- The type and intensity of rehabilitation
- The person's support system

When can rehabilitation begin?

Rehabilitation should begin as soon as possible after a stroke, within 1 or 2 days. The sooner treatment starts, the better the chances of recovery.

In some cases, rehabilitation may begin while the person is still in the hospital. In others, it may start after being discharged.

How long does stroke rehabilitation take?

The amount of time it takes to recover from a stroke varies for each individual and ranges from weeks to years. Some people may recover fully, while others face lifelong changes and disabilities.

However, with proper rehabilitation and support, many people can lead fulfilling, independent lives.

What are the stages of stroke recovery?

Recovery from a stroke is a gradual process that looks different for each person. Doctors use stages to measure stroke recovery. In stage 1, a person is unable to move their muscles. By stage 6, muscle movement is almost as before the stroke.

Physical therapist Signe Brunnstrom developed a tool for charting a person's progress to recovery. It breaks the recovery process into six stages with clear identifying factors.

Stroke recovery is a complicated process that can take months or years. Typically, the most significant improvements occur in the first 3–6 months.

Brunnstrom stages of recovery

Physical therapist Signe Brunnstrom developed the Brunnstrom Stages of Stroke Recovery in the 1960s.

The Brunnstrom stages describe the development of the ability to move and the reorganization of the brain after a stroke. This approach allows people who have had a stroke and their doctors to check the progress of their recovery.

The six stages are as follows:

Stage 1: Flaccidity

During the first stage, a person is unable to move their muscles, and they may feel limp and floppy.

Stage 2: Onset of spasticity

A person's muscles may now tighten involuntarily in response to a stimulus, such as a prod with a finger. However, the person may also have difficulty relaxing their muscles.

Stage 3: Increased spasticity

Some of the person's muscles begin to tighten. It may be even harder to relax the muscles.

However, a person may now have voluntary control over some of the basic muscle groups to manage limb movement, known as limb synergies.

Stage 4: Decreased spasticity

During this stage, involuntary muscle tightening decreases. The brain gets better at sending signals to specific muscles to move them voluntarily.

Stage 5: Increased complex voluntary movements

With involuntary muscle tightening now at a minimum, a person becomes more capable of performing complex muscle movements voluntarily.

Stage 6: Spasticity disappears, and coordination returns

A person's control of their movements almost fully returns to typical function. Involuntary muscle tightening disappears, and the person's movements become more coordinated.

Recovery timeline

Stroke recovery can happen quickly, or it may take some time. It depends on the individual's unique condition and circumstances.

A person who has had a stroke usually experiences the most significant improvements in their condition within the first 3–6 months. However, the authors of a 2019 study in the Journal of Neurophysiology found that people could see improvements even beyond 12 months.

On this basis, they recommend the revision of clinical guidelines for stroke rehabilitation.

Factors that can affect a person's recovery include:

• The part of the brain the stroke affected

• How much of the brain the stroke affected

• The person's motivation

• The level of support a person has

• The quantity and quality of their rehabilitation

• The person's health before the stroke

Possible setbacks

Various factors can affect the success of a person's rehabilitation from a stroke. Complications that may slow this progress include:

• swelling of the brain

• pneumonia due to difficulty moving or swallowing

• a urinary tract infection due to having a catheter fitted following the loss of bladder control

• Abnormal electrical activity in the brain causing seizures

• Clinical depression

• Bed sores

• Shortening of arm or leg muscles due to a reduced ability to move the limbs

• Shoulder pain due to the corresponding arm pulling on the shoulder because of weakness or paralysis

• Blood clots that form in the leg veins due to immobility from the stroke, known as deep vein thrombosis.

A person who has had a stroke is also at increased risk of having another one. According to the Centers for Disease Control and Prevention (CDC), a person who has had a stroke has a 25% chance of having another stroke within 5 years.

Some people also have what is known as a mini-stroke. This is called a transient ischemic attack (TIA), and it is a temporary disruption of the blood flow to a part of the brain. A person who has had a TIA may have as much as a 17% chance of having a stroke within 90 days. Their risk is highest during the first week.

Spontaneous recovery

The brain is an amazing organ that can reorganize its cells, molecules, and systems to help it recover from a stroke. This part of a person's rehabilitation is known as "spontaneous recovery."

Spontaneous recovery will vary from person to person, but it is not usually enough to return to pre-stroke wellness. However, in combination with available stroke rehabilitation therapies, spontaneous recovery is an important factor in restoring the function of injured but surviving brain tissue.

Outlook

Although full recovery from a stroke is possible, some people develop long-term disabilities. The type of disability depends on which part of the brain the stroke affected.

There are five main types of disability following a stroke:

• Problems controlling movement: Paralysis or weakness, usually on one side of the body, can cause problems with swallowing, posture, walking, and balance. Doctors may refer to one-sided paralysis as hemiplegia and one-sided weakness as hemiparesis.

• Sensory problems: A person may lose the ability to feel things such as touch, pain, and temperature. People may also lose bladder or bowel control and experience chronic pain due to being unable to move a joint properly.

• Problems with language: People may have difficulty speaking, writing, or understanding.

• Thinking and memory problems: The possible symptoms include a shortened attention span, short-term memory deficits, and the loss of the ability to plan, learn new tasks, or perform complex mental activities.

• Emotional disturbances: People may experience fear, anxiety, frustration, anger, sadness, or grief due to the loss of physical and mental function. Alongside the physical effects of brain injury, this can lead to clinical depression and personality changes.

The CDC says that if a person arrives at the emergency room within 3 hours of their first stroke symptom, they often have less disability after the stroke than people who did not receive care until later. For this reason, it is essential to seek prompt medical attention.

What are the risk factors for stroke?

Stroke has many risk factors, including health conditions and lifestyle habits. Understanding the different risk factors for a stroke can help prevent one from occurring.

According to the Centers for Disease Control and Prevention (CDC), every 40 seconds, a person in the United States has a stroke.

This article will cover the risk factors for a stroke.

Lifestyle and behaviors

The following lifestyle factors can increase the risk of stroke.

A lack of physical activity

If people do not exercise, they may develop health conditions that increase the risk of stroke, such as:

• high blood pressure

- high cholesterol

- obesity

- diabetes

Less healthy eating habits

To help lower the risk of stroke, a person should avoid eating a diet that is high in:

- salt

- saturated fats

- trans fats

- cholesterol

High stress levels

A 2022 study found that people with high blood pressure and persistently high levels of psychological stress had an increased risk of experiencing their first stroke or first ischemic stroke.

The authors state that they did not find a significant association between stress and hemorrhagic stroke.

Smoking

Smoking can increase a person's risk of stroke by 12% for every 5 cigarettes they smoke per day.

Tobacco smoke contains many harmful chemicals. According to the CDC, tobacco use increases the risk of stroke in the following ways:

• Smoking can cause damage to the blood vessels and heart.

• Nicotine can raise a person's blood pressure.

• Carbon monoxide reduces the amount of oxygen that the blood can carry.

Drinking too much alcohol

Drinking too much alcohol can raise a person's blood pressure and increase the levels of triglycerides in the blood. This can increase the risk of stroke.

The CDC suggests that females should not consume more than one alcoholic drink per day and males should not consume more than two per day.

Obesity

Obesity has associations with higher levels of low-density lipoprotein (LDL), or "bad" cholesterol, and another type of cholesterol called triglycerides.

It can also:

• decrease levels of high-density lipoprotein (HDL), which people sometimes call "good" cholesterol

• increase blood pressure

• increase the risk of diabetes

High blood pressure

The American Heart Associationstates that most people who have had a stroke also have high blood pressure, or hypertension. High blood pressure can damage the arteries and may cause them to clog or burst more easily.

A typical blood pressure level is 120/80 millimeters of mercury (mm Hg).

A person may be able to lower their blood pressure through lifestyle habits such as exercising regularly.

High cholesterol

In addition to monitoring their blood pressure, a person should ask a healthcare professional to check their blood cholesterol levels. A person with a total cholesterol level above 200 milligrams per deciliter (mg/dL) or an LDL level above 100 mg/dL has a condition called hyperlipidemia. A person with high cholesterol is at risk of buildup in their arteries called plaque. As plaque builds over time, it can reduce the space inside the arteries. Without treatment, this can block the blood flow from the heart to the brain, causing a stroke.

Heart disease

Heart conditions such as coronary artery disease can increase a person's risk of stroke. This is because plaque can build up in the arteries, blocking the blood flow to the brain.

Other heart conditions that can increase the risk of stroke include:

• Heart valve defects

• Irregular heartbeat

• Enlarged heart chambers

Diabetes

People with type 1 and type 2 diabetes have an increased risk of stroke.

Type 1 diabetes can damage a person's blood vessels as a result of increased blood glucose.

Many people with type 2 diabetes have other health conditions that can increase their risk of stroke, such as high cholesterol.

There is no cure for type 1 diabetes. However, people with risk factors for type 2 diabetes may be able to prevent it.

Sickle cell disease

Although this condition can affect anyone, it typically affects Black children.

The "sickled" shape of red blood cells in people with sickle cell disease means that the cells often clump together. The cells can then form clots, which may block blood vessels.

If a clot moves to the brain, a stroke can occur. This can also damage blood vessels, causing a bleed in the brain.

Risk factors a person is not able to change

Genetics, family history, age, and sex can all contribute to a person's risk of stroke, according to the CDC:

• Age: A stroke can happen at any age, but the risk increases with age. The chance of having a stroke doubles every 10 years after age 55.

• Sex: Stroke appears to be more common in females. Pregnancy and the use of birth control pills may be contributing factors.

• Family history and genetics: Genetics may play a role in conditions that contribute to the risk of stroke, such as high blood pressure and sickle cell disease. A person's family health history can be useful in understanding their risk of stroke.

Race

Black, American Indian, Native American, or Hispanic people are more likely to experience a stroke than white people.

The American Stroke Association states that Black Americans have the highest prevalence of stroke. The reasons are not clear, but two-thirds of Black Americans have at least one risk factor for stroke. The authors of a 2021 study on the association between race and the prevalence of stroke in Mississippi note that the following factors may play a role:

• socioeconomic disparities

• a lack of access to healthcare

• a lack of access to health insurance

Can vertigo indicate a stroke?

Vertigo can sometimes be a symptom of a stroke. However, it will typically occur alongside other symptoms. More common stroke symptoms include face drooping, vision changes, or sudden difficulty talking or walking.

Vertigo is a medical condition in which a person experiences a sensation of spinning or that their surroundings are spinning around them. This feeling can be disorienting and may be due to issues related to the inner ear or brain.

A stroke occurs from an interruption or reduction of blood supply to part of the brain, preventing brain tissue from getting oxygen and nutrients. This can result in the sudden death of brain cells.

Symptoms of a stroke may include sudden numbness, confusion, weakness, a severe headache, or trouble speaking, seeing, or walking. Strokes require immediate medical attention as they can lead to serious brain damage or death.

This article explains whether vertigo can indicate a stroke and when someone should contact a doctor about either condition.

Is vertigo a sign of a stroke?

Vertigo can occur during a brain stem stroke. However, it will typically occur alongside other symptoms, such as:

• difficulty speaking

• weakness or numbness on one side of the body

• vision problems, such as double vision

• a severe headache

• a decreased level of consciousness

Vertigo may also occur due to a cerebellar stroke, which can cause other symptoms, such as nausea, slurred speech, vision problems, and difficulty walking.

On its own, vertigo is not usually a sign of stroke.

What else causes vertigo?

Other potential causes of vertigo include:

• Benign paroxysmal positional vertigo (BPPV): This is the most common cause of vertigo and occurs when tiny calcium particles gather together in the canals of the inner ear, disrupting signals to the brain.

• Certain medications: Some medications can cause vertigo as a side effect.

• Meniere disease: This involves an accumulation of fluid and changing pressure in the ear, leading to episodes of vertigo, tinnitus, and hearing loss.

• Migraine: Some people with migraine experiencevertigo as a symptom, even without a headache.

• Vestibular neuritis or labyrinthitis: This is an inner ear problem usually relatedTrusted Sourceto an infection that causes inflammation around the nerves that help the body sense balance.

• Other medical conditions: Less commonly, vertigo can be a symptom of more serious medical conditions, such as a brain tumor or multiple sclerosis.

Signs of a stroke

Recognizing the signs of a stroke is critical for timely medical intervention, which can significantly improve outcomes. Common signs of a stroke include:

• sudden confusion, which may include difficulty understanding speech or trouble expressing oneself

• facial drooping

• numbness or weakness, particularly on one side of the body

• difficulty walking or trouble with coordination

• difficulty speaking, such as slurred speech

• sudden vision changes in one or both eyes

• a sudden, severe headache with no apparent cause

Treatment

Learn about the treatment options for a stroke and vertigo below.

Stroke

The immediate treatment for a stroke depends on the type of stroke a person is having.

An ischemic stroke occurs due to a blockage of blood vessels supplying blood to the brain. Its treatment involves medications to dissolve clots and restore blood flow to the brain.

The first-line option is tissue plasminogen activator (tPA), which requires administration within 3 hours from the onset of symptoms for effectiveness.

Hemorrhagic stroke occurs due to bleeding in the brain. Treatment aims to control bleeding and reduce pressure in the brain. Surgery may be necessary to repair damaged blood vessels or relieve pressure.

Brain stem strokes can occur due to clots or a hemorrhage, so treatment will depend on its origin.

After the stroke, treatment steps may include:

• post-stroke rehabilitation, such as:

• physical therapy

• occupational therapy

• speech therapy

• medications to manage blood pressure

• lifestyle changes, such as:

• a balanced diet

• regular exercise

• quitting or stopping smoking

• limiting or avoiding alcohol

Vertigo

Treatment for vertigo may include:

• Medications: Depending on the cause, medications may relieve symptoms, such as nausea or motion sickness. For Meniere disease, doctors may prescribe diuretics.

• Physical therapy: Vestibular rehabilitation is a type of therapy designed to alleviate symptoms of vertigo. Exercises aim to improve balance and reduce dizziness.

• Canalith repositioning maneuvers: For BPPV, a doctor can perform specific head and body movements, such as the Epley maneuver, to move calcium deposits out of the ear canal into an inner ear chamber.

• Lifestyle adjustments: Doctors may advise people to make adjustments to reduce the risk of falls and manage triggers for vertigo.

When to contact a doctor

People should seek emergency medical help if they experience vertigo alongside any sudden symptoms of a stroke, including:

• numbness or weakness in the face, arms, or legs, especially on one side of the body

• confusion, trouble speaking, or difficulty understanding speech

• trouble seeing in one or both eyes

• trouble walking, dizziness, a loss of balance, or a lack of coordination

• a severe headache with no known cause

Vertigo alone is not a likely indicator of stroke. However, people can speak with a healthcare professional to identify the underlying cause and learn about their treatment options.

What tests might a doctor order for stroke?

Doctors can perform various tests to determine whether someone is having a stroke and to diagnose the type. Tests may include physical exams, blood tests, heart tests, and imaging, among others.

Strokes occur when an area of the brain stops receiving blood and oxygen, causing several symptoms, such as slurred speech or weakness on one side of the body.

There are two main types of stroke. An ischemic stroke is the most prevalent type, but people can also experience hemorrhagic strokes. Accurate diagnosis is crucial for providing appropriate treatment.

Doctors can use a combination of medical tests to determine what type of stroke a person has. Still, if the healthcare professional suspects someone is having a stroke according to symptoms alone, then they will prioritize treatment over diagnostic tests.

This article reviews the tests doctors use to diagnose stroke and the steps they usually take after diagnosis.

Physical exam

Doctors perform a physical exam to evaluate the symptoms a person presents with and give them a score.

The National Institutes of Health Stroke Scale (NIHSS) gauges the presence and severity of a stroke according to the final score.

The NIHSS uses the following parameters to determine this score:

• the ability to answer questions about location and time

• eye movement and visual acuity, which tests how the eye differentiates shapes and details of objects

• facial movement or paralysis

• the ability to move legs and arms

• sensation to touch

• the ability to perform physical instructions

• level of consciousness

• the ability to understand written and verbal communication

• the ability to speak and clarity

Read about what to expect with physical exams.

Heart and blood tests

Doctors may order blood and heart tests for a person they suspect is having a stroke.

These tests may not indicate the location or presence of a stroke. However, they can provide important information about potential triggers, such as a blood clotting complication.

Some tests doctors may order include:

• a complete blood count to look at the different markers in the blood

• tests that assess for electrolyte issues

• tests that assess for clotting issues

• tests that assess muscle damage to the heart

• an EKG to measure the electrical activity of the heart muscle and help diagnose atrial fibrillation or a previous heart attack

Imaging tests

Doctors may use a combination of imaging tests in their diagnostic workup.

These tests include:

• CT scan: A CT scan of the brain — also known as cranial CT scan — can determine if there is any bleeding or damage in the brain.

• MRI: This test can show if there are any tissue changes in the brain.

• Other imaging tests: This may include a PET or a subtraction angiography to check for any narrowing of blood vessels in the neck, aneurysms, or any other atypical formations in the brain that may have led to the stroke. Specialized tests such as CT angiography and CT perfusion may also be useful.

These tests produce images of the tissues and blood vessels in the brain, making it easier to spot bleeding, clots, or other potential issues that may have led to stroke. Imaging can also help determine the type of stroke that has occurred, including its location and extent.

Lumbar puncture

A lumbar puncture — also known as a spinal tap — may help when a doctor suspects a person is experiencing subarachnoid hemorrhage, a type of hemorrhagic stroke.

To perform a lumbar puncture, a healthcare professional will collect fluid from a person's spine using a needle. They will then test the fluid, looking for substances relating to damaged blood cells.

Next steps after tests

After diagnosing the type, extent, and location of the stroke, doctors will use this information to devise a short-term or long-term treatment plan. If they strongly suspect the person is currently having a stroke, they will prioritize treatment over testing.

Timing is crucial as the brain can develop permanent damage, which may lead to disability when there is a disruption or blockage of blood flow in the body, even for just a few minutes. If a person feels like they are experiencing stroke symptoms, they need immediate medical attention.

Contrastingly, from other cells in the human body, once the tissues and cells in the brain die due to the lack of oxygen, it is not possible to repair or restore them, leading to permanent damage. The primary aim of the treatment is to restore the blood flow to the brain as soon as possible to minimize and reduce the risk of further brain damage.

Doctors can use a combination of surgery and medications to treat a stroke, depending on its type.

Generally, treating ischemic strokes involves administering a tissue plasminogen activator (tpA). This helps break up blood clots that may be affecting blood flow to the brain. The sooner treatment starts, the better.

If a person cannot have tpA anti-platelet or blood-thinning medications, such as aspirin or clopidogrel (Plavix), may be necessary.

Doctors may recommend anticoagulant drugs, such as warfarin (Coumadin), to people to prevent future strokes.

If a person experiences a hemorrhagic stroke, treatment typically focuses on:

• stopping the bleeding

• reducing the pressure inside the skull

• preventing and managing high blood pressure and seizures

Doctors can typically achieve these goals by prescribing medications, such as saline solutions and mannitol (Osmitrol), or performing surgery.

A person may also receive additional care, such as:

• fluids

• breathing support

• compression therapy

• insertion of a feeding tube as it may be difficult for a person to swallow

• skin care to prevent skin irritation and the development of sores

• rehabilitation plans to relearn how to swallow, speak, and walk if a stroke has affected any of these

The Ultimate Stroke Diet Recipes for Beginners

Mediterranean Bowl

1. Calories 488 Per Serving

2. Protein 17g Per Serving

3. Fiber 12g Per Serving

Ingredients

Servings: 4

Serving Size: 1 1/2 cups

Ingredients

• 1 cup uncooked whole grain sorghum

Dressing

• 1/4 cup olive, canola or corn oil

• 2 tablespoons lime juice (from 1/2 medium lime)

• 1 tablespoon chopped cilantro

• 1 garlic clove, minced

- 1/2 to 1 teaspoon Dijon mustard (lowest sodium available)
- 1/4 to 1/2 teaspoon ground cumin
- 1/4 teaspoon salt
- 1/4 teaspoon pepper
- 1 cup grape or cherry tomatoes (about ½ pint), halved
- 1 15.5-ounce can no-salt-added chickpeas, cannellini beans, red kidney or black beans (rinsed and drained)
- 1/2 cup jarred roasted red bell peppers
- 1/2 cup frozen shelled edamame, thawed
- 1/2 cup chopped cucumber
- 1/2 cup green onions (about 4 medium), green parts only, chopped
- 1/4 cup fat-free feta cheese
- 1/2 medium avocado, pitted and sliced into 8 slices

Directions

- Prepare the sorghum using the package directions, omitting the salt.
- Meanwhile, in a small bowl, whisk together the dressing ingredients. Set aside.

• In a medium bowl, stir together the tomatoes, beans, bell peppers, edamame, cucumber and green onions. Stir in the cooked sorghum. Pour the dressing all over, stirring to coat.

• Put the sorghum mixture into serving bowls. Sprinkle with the feta. Top with the avocado slices.

Sweet and Sour Pork Fried Rice

1. Calories 490 Per Serving

2. Protein 31g Per Serving

3. Fiber 6g Per Serving

Ingredients

Servings: 4

Serving Size: 1 1/2 cups

Marinade Ingredients

• 1 tablespoon soy sauce (lowest sodium available)

• 1 tablespoon plain rice vinegarOR

• 1 tablespoon dry sherry

• 1 teaspoon cornstarch

• 1 pound pork tenderloin, all visible fat discarded, cut into 3/4-inch cubes

Sauce Ingredients

• 1/2 cup fat-free, low-sodium chicken broth

• 1/2 cup all-fruit apricot spread

• 2 tablespoons plain rice vinegarOR

• 2 tablespoons white wine vinegar

• 1 tablespoon soy sauce (lowest sodium available)

• Cooking spray

• 2 large eggs, lightly beaten with a fork

• 1 teaspoon canola or corn oil

• 2 to 3 teaspoons crushed red pepper flakes

• 1 medium red bell pepper, cut into 1-inch pieces

• 1 medium carrot, diced

• 3 cups cooked brown rice (cold preferred)

• 1 8-ounce can pineapple chunks in their own juice, drained

• 1 cup frozen green peas, thawed

• 4 medium green onions, sliced

Directions

• In a large glass dish, whisk together the marinade ingredients. Add the pork, turning to coat. Cover and refrigerate for 10 minutes to 8 hours, turning occasionally.

• Meanwhile, in a small bowl, whisk together the sauce ingredients. Set aside.

• When the pork is done marinating, heat a wok or large skillet over medium-high heat. Remove from the heat and lightly spray with cooking spray (being careful not to spray near a gas flame). Cook the eggs for 1 to 2 minutes, stirring frequently, until scrambled. Break up into pieces. Transfer to a plate.

• Carefully wipe the wok with paper towels. Heat the oil over high heat, swirling to coat the bottom. Cook the pork with the marinade and the red pepper flakes for 5 minutes, or until the pork is no longer pink on the outside and tender, stirring frequently. Cook the bell pepper and carrots for 2 to 3 minutes, or until tender-crisp, stirring frequently.

• Stir in the rice, pineapple, peas, green onions, reserved broth mixture and reserved egg pieces. Reduce the heat to medium. Cook for 3 to 5 minutes, or until the mixture is warmed through, stirring occasionally to break up the rice.

Yellow Squash Soup (Ogwissimanabo)

1. Calories 30 Per Serving

2. Protein 1g Per Serving

3. Fiber 1g Per Serving

Ingredients

Servings: 4

• 4 cups water

• 2 medium yellow squash (chopped)

• 1 small onion (chopped)

• 1/8 teaspoon salt

• 1 tablespoon honey

• cucumber

• 1/4 teaspoon garlic powder

• 1/2 teaspoon black pepper

Directions

• In a medium pot, bring water to a boil.

• Add squash, onion, salt, and honey.

• Reduce heat to medium, cover, and simmer for 25 minutes.

• Transfer the mixture to a bowl, add cucumbers and mash into a paste.

• Return past to pot, add garlic and pepper and simmer over medium heat for 10-15 minutes.

Quick Tips

1. Tip: Engage the kids--mashing the squash mixture and cucumbers into a paste is a great way to get the kids involved--consider letting the mixture cool slightly before letting small children mash.

Tandoori Chicken with Brown Rice

1. Calories 243 Per Serving
2. Protein 28g Per Serving
3. Fiber 1g Per Serving

Ingredients

Servings: 4

• 1 lb. boneless, skinless chicken breasts or tenderloins (all visible fat discarded)

- 1/4 cup fresh lemon juiceOR

- 1/4 cup jarred lime juice

- 1/2 cup plain, fat-free yogurt

- 3 clove fresh garlic (minced)OR

- 3 tsp. jarred, minced garlic

- 1 tsp. ground cumin

- 1/2 tsp. paprika

- 1/2 tsp. turmeric

- 1/2 tsp. ground ginger

- 1/4 tsp. pepper

- 1 cup instant brown rice

Directions

• Preheat oven to 400 degrees.

• Place chicken in a 9x9 baking dish and pierce chicken pieces with a fork all over.

• In a small bowl, whisk together lemon juice, yogurt, garlic, cumin, paprika, turmeric, ginger and pepper.

• Add mixture to chicken, turning to coat, let stand 20 minutes (or refrigerate overnight). Bake for 15 minutes, turn chicken and bake 15 minutes more.

• While chicken bakes prepare rice to package instructions.

• Serve chicken over rice.

Athenian Beef Meatloaf with Cucumber-Yogurt Sauce

1. Calories 198 Per Serving
2. Protein 28g Per Serving
3. Fiber

Ingredients

Servings: 8

Serving Size: 1/8 slice meatloaf, 1/4 c sauce

• 2 lbs ground beef (96% lean)

• 1 cup soft bread crumbs

• 3/4 cup finely chopped onion

• 1/2 cup 1% low-fat milk

• 1 large egg

• 1 tablespoon plus 1-1/2 teaspoons dried Greek seasoning, divided

• 1/2 teaspoon salt

• 1 cup plain, low-fat Greek yogurt

• 1/2 cup diced cucumber

Directions

• Preheat oven to 350°F. Combine Ground Beef, bread crumbs, onion, milk, egg, 1 tablespoon Greek seasoning and salt in large bowl, mixing lightly but thoroughly.

• Shape beef mixture into 10 x 4-inch loaf on rack in broiler pan. Bake in 350°F oven 1-1/4 to 1-1/2 hours, until instant-read thermometer inserted into center registers 160°F.

• Meanwhile, combine yogurt, cucumber and remaining 1-1/2 teaspoons Greek seasoning in medium bowl. Season with salt, as desired. Set aside.

• Let meatloaf stand 10 minutes; cut into 8 slices. Serve with cucumber-yogurt sauce.

Quick Tips

1. Tip: To make soft bread crumbs, place torn bread in food processor or blender container. Cover; pulse on and off, to form fine crumbs. One and one-half slices make about 1 cup crumbs.

2. Tip: Cooking times are for fresh or thoroughly thawed ground beef. Ground beef should be cooked to an internal

temperature of 160°F. Color is not a reliable indicator of ground beef doneness.

Heart-Healthy Nicoise Salad

1. Calories 177 Per Serving
2. Protein 12g Per Serving
3. Fiber

Ingredients

Servings: 6

Serving Size   approx. 2 C

• 1 1/2 - 2 pounds potatoes, peeled (if desired) and cut into 1/2-inch cubes; approx. 4-5 cup

• 1/2 cup bottled, reduced-calorie ranch salad dressing

• 1-2 teaspoons curry powder (to taste)

• 2 6-ounce cans tuna (packed in water), drained

• 1 cup green onions (chopped)

• 1/2 cup pitted olives (black or green), chopped

• 4 - 6 cups washed and drained mixed salad greens

• 6 plum tomatoes, quartered lengthwise

• 4 hard boiled egg whites, quartered lengthwise

Directions

• Over high heat, bring a large pot of water to boil. Add cubed potatoes; return to boiling and simmer 5 minutes or until tender, but firm. Drain potatoes and set aside or refrigerate.

• In a large bowl, mix together ranch dressing and curry powder to taste. Stir in tuna, green onions and olives. Gently stir in potatoes.

• To serve, arrange greens on a platter (or on individual dishes), top with potato mixture, then garnish with tomatoes and eggs.

Couscous with Chickpeas

1. Calories 216 Per Serving

2. Protein 10g Per Serving

3. Fiber 7g Per Serving

Ingredients

Servings: 6

Serving Size   1 1/2 cups

• 2/3 cup uncooked whole-wheat couscous

• 1 1/3 cups boiling water

• Juice of 1 medium lemon

• 1 15-ounce can no-salt-added chickpeas, rinsed and drained

• 1 large bell pepper (red, yellow, or orange preferred), cut into 1/4-inch pieces

• 2 tablespoons plus 1 1/2 teaspoons dried basil

• 2 tablespoons plus 1 1/2 teaspoons dried parsley

• 2 medium garlic cloves, mincedOR

• 1 teaspoon bottled minced garlic

• 1 tablespoon plus 1 teaspoon canola, corn, or olive oil

• 1/4 cup fat-free crumbled feta cheeseOR

• 1/4 cup shredded Parmesan cheese

Directions

• Pour the couscous in a large, heatproof bowl. Pour in the water and lemon juice. Let stand for 15 minutes. Fluff with a fork.

• In a large bowl, stir together the couscous and chickpeas.

• Stir in the bell peppers, basil, parsley, and garlic.

• Drizzle with the oil. Sprinkle with the cheese.

• Serve at room temperature or refrigerate, covered, for 2 to 12 hours.

Tuna Stir-Fry

1. Calories 236 Per Serving
2. Protein 24g Per Serving
3. Fiber 5g Per Serving

Ingredients

Servings: 4

• 2 cups cooked brown rice

• Cooking spray

• 1/2 medium onion, chopped

• 2 medium garlic cloves, mincedOR

• 1 teaspoon jarred minced garlic

• 1 16-ounce package frozen stir-fry vegetables

• 2 4.5-ounce cans or 2 2.6-ounce pouches very low sodium albacore tuna, packed in water, drained and flaked

- 2 tablespoons soy sauce (lowest sodium available)

- Juice of 1 medium lemon

- 1 teaspoon honey

Directions

- Prepare the rice using the package directions, omitting the salt and margarine.

- Lightly spray a large skillet with cooking spray. Cook the onion, garlic, and stir-fry vegetables over medium-high heat for 5 minutes, or until the vegetables are tender-crisp.

- Stir in the tuna, soy sauce, lemon juice, and honey. Cook for 2 to 3 minutes, or until the tuna is heated through.

- Serve over the rice.

Avocado Salsa

1. Calories 108 Per Serving

2. Protein 3g Per Serving

3. Fiber

Ingredients

Servings: 16

• 16 6-inch corn tortillas, each cut into 6 wedges

• 1/8 tsp salt and 1/8 tsp salt and 1/4 tsp salt (divided use)

• 1/2 can no-salt-added black beans (rinsed, drained)

• 1 medium cucumber (peeled, seeded, finely chopped)

• 1 small green bell pepper (finely chopped)

• 1 medium rib of celery (finely chopped)

• 2-3 tablespoon snipped, fresh cilantro

• 2 tablespoon fresh lime juice

• 1/8 teaspoon crushed red pepper flakes

• 2 medium avocados (diced)

Directions

• Preheat the oven to 350°F.

• On a large baking sheet, arrange half the tortilla wedges in a single layer. Bake for 10 minutes, or until lightly golden. Sprinkle with 1/8 teaspoon salt. Transfer to a serving bowl. Repeat with the remaining tortilla wedges and the remaining 1/8 teaspoon salt.

• Meanwhile, in a medium serving bowl, stir together the beans, cucumber, bell pepper, celery, cilantro, lime juice, the final 1/4 teaspoon salt and red pepper flakes. Using a rubber scraper, gently fold in the avocados. Serve with the tortilla wedges.

Quick Tips

1. Tip: Serving size 1/4 cup salsa and 6 chips

Black Bean Soup

1. Calories 245 Per Serving

2. Protein 15g Per Serving

3. Fiber 11g Per Serving

Ingredients

Servings: 4

• Cooking spray

• 1 medium onion, diced

• 1 medium fresh jalapeño, seeds and ribs discarded, chopped

• 1 tablespoon minced garlic

• 2 teaspoons ground cumin

• 2 15.5-ounce cans no-salt-added black beans, undrained

• 1 14.5-ounce can no-salt-added diced tomatoes, undrained

• 1 cup fat-free, low-sodium chicken broth

• 1/4 cup chopped fresh cilantro (optional)

Directions

• Lightly spray a large pot with cooking spray.

• Cook the onion over medium-high heat for 5 minutes, or until very soft, stirring frequently. Stir in the jalapeño, garlic, and cumin. Cook for 1 minute.

• Stir in the beans with liquid. Lightly mash them using a potato masher or fork. Stir in the tomatoes with liquid and broth. Reduce the heat to medium. Simmer, covered, for 15 minutes.

• Serve the soup topped with the cilantro.

Quick Tips

1. Tip: To save money, buy the store brand of canned beans with the least amount of sodium. Look for "no-salt-added" and "reduced-sodium" options. An unopened can of beans can last up to two years in a pantry, so stock up when they go on sale.

2. Keep it Healthy: Be sure to shop for no-salt-added or reduced-sodium canned beans (for all types) since there's a big difference in the varieties. For example, a half-cup serving of regular canned beans contains between 350 and 565 milligrams of sodium. By comparison, the same quantity in the reduced-sodium version has about 220 milligrams, and the no-salt-added version has even less, only 15 milligrams.

Vegetable and Goat Cheese Phyllo Pie

1. Calories 230 Per Serving
2. Protein 15g Per Serving
3. Fiber 5g per serving

Ingredients

Servings: 4

• Cooking spray

• 1 Tbsp. olive oil (extra virgin preferred)

• 4-5 medium green onions (about 1 cup), chopped

• 2 medium zucchini (thinly sliced)

- 10 oz. frozen, chopped spinach (thawed, squeezed dry)
- 1/4 cup chopped, fresh parsley
- 2 Tbsp. chopped, fresh mint
- 2 medium garlic cloves (minced)
- 1 cup fat-free evaporated milk
- 1/2 cup egg substitute
- 1/4 tsp. pepper
- 1/8 tsp. ground nutmeg
- 6 phyllo dough sheets (each 14 x 9 inches), thawed
- 1 1/2 oz. soft goat cheese

Directions

- Preheat the oven to 375°F. Lightly spray a 9-inch pie pan with cooking spray. Set aside.
- In a large nonstick skillet, heat the oil over medium heat, swirling to coat the bottom. Cook the green onions for 2 minutes, or until softened, stirring frequently.
- Stir in the zucchini. Cook for 4 minutes, or until beginning to brown, stirring frequently.
- Stir in the spinach, parsley, mint, and garlic. Cook for 2 minutes, stirring frequently.

• In a small bowl, whisk together the evaporated milk, egg substitute, pepper, and nutmeg. Set aside.

• Working quickly and keeping the unused phyllo covered with damp paper towels to prevent drying, place one sheet of phyllo in the pie pan, gently pressing on the bottom and side of the pan, letting the ends overhang the pan. Repeat with the remaining phyllo, placing the sheets in a crisscross pattern.

• Spoon the green onion mixture over the phyllo. Pour in the milk mixture, swirling if needed to cover the surface. Dot with the cheese.

• Fold the ends of the phyllo toward the center of the pan, leaving a circle of the filling showing. Lightly spray the phyllo with cooking spray. Gently press the phyllo on the filling so the phyllo will hold its shape.

• Bake for 30 to 40 minutes, or until golden. Transfer to a cooling rack and let cool for 15 minutes. Cut into wedges. Serve warm.

Quick Tips

1. Tip: Serving size 1 wedge

Creole Steak with Jambalaya Rice

1. Calories 338 Per Serving
2. Protein 29g Per Serving
3. Fiber 4.7g Per Serving

Ingredients

Servings: 4

Serving Size1/4 cup rice mix, 1/2 cup sliced steak

• 1 1/2 cups cooked brown rice

• 1 cup chopped celery

• 2 1/2 teaspoons Creole seasoning, divided

• 1 cup chopped green bell pepper

• 1 cup chopped onion

• 1 lb sirloin tip steaks, cut-1/4 inch thick

• 1 can (14 1/2 ounces) no salt added diced tomatoes

• 2 tablespoons vegetable oil (divided)

Directions

• Heat 1 tablespoon oil over medium heat in 3-quart saucepan until hot. Add onion, celery, bell pepper and 1 teaspoon Creole seasoning; cook 8 to 10 minutes or until vegetables are crisp-tender, stirring occasionally.

• Stir in tomatoes and rice. Cover and continue cooking 2 to 4 minutes or until heated through, stirring occasionally. Keep warm.

• Meanwhile, press remaining 1-1/2 teaspoons Creole seasoning evenly onto beef steaks. Heat 1-1/2 teaspoons oil in large nonstick skillet over medium-high heat until hot. Cooking in batches, place steaks in skillet (do not overcrowd) and cook 1 to 3 minutes for medium rare (145°F) doneness, turning once. (Do not overcook.) Remove from skillet; keep warm. Repeat with remaining steaks and oil.

• Serve steaks topped with rice mixture.

Cajun-Creole Smothered Steaks

1. Calories 225 Per Serving
2. Protein 28g Per Serving
3. Fiber 3g Per Serving

Ingredients

Servings: 2

Serving Size: 3 ounces steak and 1/2 C vegetables

• 2 teaspoons salt-free Cajun-Creole seasoning blend

• 2 teaspoons olive oil

• 1/2 14.5-ounce can no-salt-added diced tomatoes, undrained (about 1 cup)

• 1/4 cup water

• 1/2 medium green bell pepper (chopped)

• 1/2 medium rib of celery, cut into 1/2-inch slices

• 2 tablespoons chopped onion

• 1 medium garlic clove (minced)

• 1/4 teaspoon salt

• 2 eye-of-round steaks (about 4 ounces each), all visible fat discarded

Directions

• Sprinkle the seasoning blend over both sides of the steaks.

• In a medium skillet, heat the oil over medium-high heat, swirling to coat the bottom. Cook the steaks for 2 minutes on each side, or until browned. Transfer to a plate.

• In the same skillet, stir together the tomatoes with liquid, water, bell pepper, celery, onion, garlic, and salt. Add the steaks. Spoon the sauce over the steaks. Bring to a simmer. Reduce the heat and simmer for 1 hour 15 minutes, or until tender.

Quick Tips

1. Tip: If you are pressed for time, you can serve the steaks after about 45 minutes of simmering. They should be tender enough by then, though they will be even better with the full simmering time.

Pot Roast Ratatouille and Pasta - Delicious Decisions

1. Calories 258 Per Serving
2. Protein 26g Per Serving
3. Fiber 6g Per Serving

Ingredients

Servings: 8

- olive oil spray
- 1 1/2 lb. eye-of-round roast (all visible fat discarded)
- 1/2 tsp. salt-free, all-purpose seasoning blend
- 1/4 tsp. pepper
- 10.75 oz. canned tomato puree
- 10 oz. eggplant (chopped)
- 2 medium zucchini (sliced)
- 5 medium Italian plum (Roma) tomatoes (chopped)
- 1 large onion (chopped)
- 2 medium ribs of celery, sliced
- 1 tsp. oregano or Italian seasoning, crumbled
- 1 medium garlic clove (minced)
- 1 medium dried bay leaf
- 1/4 tsp. dried basil (crumbled)
- 8 oz. dried, whole-grain pasta

Directions

- Preheat the oven to 350°F. Lightly spray a Dutch oven with olive oil spray.
- Sprinkle the roast with the seasoning blend and pepper.
- Heat the Dutch oven over medium-high heat. Brown the roast for 2 to 3 minutes on each side.

• Stir in the remaining ingredients except the pasta.

• Bake, covered, for about 2 hours, or until the roast is very tender when tested with a fork.

• Shortly before the roast is done, prepare the pasta using the package directions, omitting the salt. Drain well in a colander.

• Transfer the roast to a cutting board. Cover with aluminum foil and let stand for 10 to 15 minutes before slicing very thinly across the grain, then slicing into thin strips. Discard the bay leaf from the sauce.

• Spoon the pasta onto plates. Arrange the roast slices on the pasta. Top with the sauce.

Quick Tips

1. Tip: For maximum tenderness, don't overcook eye-of-round roast, and be sure to cut it into thin strips.

Olive Oil Mashed Potatoes

1. Calories 134 Per Serving
2. Protein 2g Per Serving

3. Fiber 3g Per Serving

Ingredients

Servings: 8

Serving Size: 1/2 cup

• 1 1/2 pounds small Yukon Gold potatoes, halved or cut into 2-inch pieces

• 6 medium garlic cloves

• 1/4 cup olive oil (extra virgin preferred)

• 1/2 teaspoon black pepper (freshly ground)

• 1/4 teaspoon salt

• 1 cup chopped green onions

Directions

• Put the potatoes, garlic, and salt in a large saucepan. Pour in enough water to cover the potatoes. Bring to a boil over high heat. Boil for 15 to 20 minutes, or until the potatoes are soft. Transfer the potatoes and garlic to a colander. Drain well. Return them to the pan.

• Using the tines of a fork, mash the potatoes and garlic, being sure to crush each piece of potato and each garlic clove.

• Add the green onions, oil, and pepper, stirring until well combined.

Meatloaf with Black-Eyed Peas

1. Calories 322 Per Serving

2. Protein 40g Per Serving

3. Fiber 7g Per Serving

4. Cost Per Serving

Ingredients

Servings: 6

Serving Size: 1 slice meat loaf and 1/2 cup black-eyed peas

• 1 medium bell pepper (any color), finely chopped

• 1 small onion, finely chopped

• 1 teaspoon canola or corn oilOR

• 1 teaspoon olive oil (extra virgin preferred)

• 1 1/2 pounds ground skinless turkey breast, extra-lean ground beef, or extra-lean ground pork

• 1/3 cup quick-cooking rolled oats

• 2 large eggs, lightly beaten using a fork

• 1 8-ounce can no-salt-added tomato sauce

• 2 tablespoons fat-free milk

• 1 tablespoon Dijon mustard (lowest sodium available)

• 1 teaspoon dried parsley

• 2 medium garlic cloves, mincedOR

• 1 teaspoon bottled minced garlic

• 1/4 teaspoon pepper

• Cooking spray

• 1 teaspoon cider vinegar2

• 15-ounce cans no-salt-added black-eyed peas, undrained

Directions

• Preheat the oven to 350°F.

• In a 9 x 5 x 3-inch glass loaf pan, stir together the bell pepper and onion. Drizzle with the oil, tossing to coat. Cover the loaf pan with a plate. Microwave on 100% (high) for 3 minutes. Allow the bell pepper mixture to cool slightly.

• In a medium bowl, using your hands or a spoon, combine the bell pepper mixture, turkey, oats, eggs, 2 tablespoons of the tomato sauce, the milk, mustard, parsley, garlic and pepper.

• Lightly spray the loaf pan with cooking spray. Shape the turkey mixture into a loaf. Place it in the pan.

• In the same medium bowl, stir together the remaining tomato sauce and the cider vinegar. Pour over the loaf.

• Bake for 50 minutes to 1 hour, or until the loaf registers 165°F (160°F for beef or pork) on an instant-read thermometer. Let stand for 5 to 10 minutes before slicing.

• Meanwhile, in a microwaveable dish, microwave the black-eyed peas with liquid on 100% power (high) for 5 minutes, or until heated through. Rinse and drain. Serve the peas with the meat loaf.

Quick Tips

1. Keep it Healthy: Many meat loaves are made with bread crumbs, which can be high in sodium, to help bind the loaf. This recipe calls for rolled oats instead, which are very low in sodium.

2. Tip: If you're in a rush or just want fun mini meat loaves for the kids, divide the turkey mixture among the cups of a standard 12-cup muffin pan. Bake for 30 minutes, or until each "muffin" registers 165°F (160°F for beef or pork) on an instant-read thermometer.

Red Beans and Rice with Corn on the Cob

1. Calories 413 Per Serving
2. Protein 15g Per Serving
3. Fiber 8g Per Serving

Ingredients

Servings: 4

Serving Size: 1 cup red beans and rice mixture and 1 ear corn

Corn on the Cob

• 4 large ears of corn, husks and silks discarded

• Butter-flavor cooking spray

• Pepper to taste (freshly ground preferred)

Red Beans and Rice

• 1 cup uncooked long-grain brown rice

• 2 teaspoons olive oil (extra virgin preferred)

• 1/2 small white onion, thinly slicedOR

• 4 medium green onions, thinly sliced

• 4 medium garlic cloves, choppedOR

• 2 teaspoons jarred minced garlic

• 1 1/2 cups cooked red beans, cooked without salt, or 1 15.5-ounce can no-salt-added red beans, kidney beans, black beans, pinto beans, or black-eyed peas, rinsed and drained

• 1/2 teaspoon salt-free Creole or Cajun seasoning blend

• 1/4 teaspoon pepper (freshly ground preferred)

Directions

Corn on the Cob

• Bring a large pot of water to a boil over high heat. Cook the corn, covered, for 5 minutes. Drain and rinse under cold water.

• Transfer the corn to a baking sheet. Gently pat dry with paper towels. Lightly spray the corn with cooking spray. Sprinkle with the pepper. Serve the corn with the red bean and rice mixture.

Red Beans and Rice

• Prepare the rice using the package directions, omitting the salt and margarine.

• Meanwhile, in a large skillet, heat the oil over medium heat, swirling to coat the bottom. Cook the onions for 2 minutes, or until soft, stirring occasionally. Stir in the garlic. Cook for 1 minute. Stir in the beans, seasoning blend, and pepper. Cook for 3 to 5 minutes, or until heated through, stirring occasionally.

• Stir the rice into the bean mixture.

Green Chile Stew

1. Calories 217 Per Serving

2. Protein 27g Per Serving

3. Fiber 2g Per Serving

Ingredients

Servings: 4

• 1 tablespoon canola oilOR

• 1 tablespoon corn oil

• 1 pound beef sirloin, round steak, or flank steak, cut into 1/2-inch cubes, all visible fat discarded

• 1 small yellow or white onion, chopped

• 2 medium garlic cloves, mincedOR

• 1 teaspoon jarred minced garlic

• 2 tablespoons whole-wheat flour

• 2 cups chopped tomatoesOR

• 1 14.5-ounce can no-salt-added diced tomatoes

• 6 fresh Hatch peppers, roasted, skinned, seeds and ribs discarded, and choppedOR

• 2 3-ounce cans diced green chiles, drained

• 1 medium fresh jalapeño or serrano pepper, seeds and ribs discarded, chopped (optional)

• 1/2 teaspoon black pepper

• 2 cups fat-free, low-sodium chicken broth

Directions

• In a large stockpot, heat the oil over medium-high heat, swirling to coat the bottom. Cook the beef for 5 minutes, or until browned on all sides, stirring occasionally.

• Cook the onion and garlic for 2 to 3 minutes, or until the onion is soft, stirring occasionally.

• Stir in the flour until well blended.

• Stir in the tomatoes, Hatch peppers, jalapeño, black pepper, and broth.

• Reduce the heat to medium low. Simmer, covered, for 1 hour.

Indian Beef Flank Steak and Rice

1. Calories 300 Per Serving

2. Protein 31g Per Serving

3. Fiber 4g Per Serving

Ingredients

Servings: 8

Serving Size about 1/2 cup beef (3 ounces cooked beef); rice blend 3/4 cup

• 1 beef Flank Steak (about 2 pounds)

• 1 cup plain, fat-free Greek yogurt

• 2 tablespoons garam masala

• 1 tablespoon garlic powder

• 1 tablespoon paprika

• 1 teaspoon salt

• 2 red onions, cut into slices (1/4 inch thick)

• 3 tablespoons water

- 3 cups cooked brown rice
- 2 cups frozen peas (cooked)

Directions

- Combine yogurt, garam masala, garlic powder, paprika and salt in small bowl. Spread 1/3 cup yogurt mixture over steak. Reserve remaining yogurt mixture for sauce. Place beef steak in food-safe plastic bag; turn steak to coat. Close bag securely and marinate in refrigerator 6 hours or as long as overnight.
- Remove steak from marinade; discard marinade. Place steak on grid over medium, ash-covered coals. Grill, covered, 11 to 16 minutes (over medium heat on preheated gas grill, covered, 16 to 21 minutes) for medium rare (145°F) to medium (160°F) doneness, turning occasionally. Meanwhile, grill onion slices, covered, 11 to 15 minutes. Remove steak from grill; let stand 3 to 5 minutes.
- Meanwhile, heat remaining sauce and water in small saucepan over medium heat 2 to 3 minutes. Cut steak lengthwise in half, then across the grain into thin slices. Cut onions into bite-sized pieces. Combine rice and peas in

large bowl. Divide rice mixture evenly among plates. Serve with beef, onions and sauce.

Slow Cooker Panang Curry with Chicken and Cauliflower Rice

1. Calories 330 Per Serving
2. Protein 32g Per Serving
3. Fiber 10g Per Serving

Ingredients

Servings 4

Cauliflower Rice

• 1 medium head cauliflower, cut into florets

• Cooking spray

• 1/4 teaspoon salt

• 1/4 teaspoon pepper

• 1/4 cup chopped fresh parsleyOR

• 2 teaspoons dried parsley (crumbled)

Garnishes (optional)

• 8 fresh basil leaves, coarsely torn

- 1 medium jalapeño, seeds and ribs discarded, sliced
- 1 medium lime, cut into 4 wedges

Curry

- 1 pound boneless, skinless chicken breasts, all visible fat discarded, cut into 1-inch cubes
- 1 medium sweet potato, peeled and cut into 1-inch cubesOR
- 1 1/2 cups butternut squash, peeled and cut into 1-inch cubes
- 1 medium onion, diced
- 3 medium garlic cloves, minced
- 1 14.5-ounce can no-salt-added diced tomatoes, undrained
- 1 cup water
- 3/4 cup unsweetened lite coconut milk
- 1 6-ounce can no-salt-added tomato paste
- 2 tablespoons low-calorie sweetener
- 2 teaspoons curry powder
- 1 teaspoon cumin
- 1 teaspoon coriander
- 1 to 2 teaspoons crushed red pepper flakes
- 1/4 cup fresh basil leaves, thinly slicedOR
- 1 tablespoon dried basil, crumbled

• 1 1/2 cups broccoli florets

Directions

• Put the chicken, sweet potato, onion, garlic, tomatoes with liquid, water, coconut milk, and tomato paste in a slow cooker.

• In a small bowl, stir together the sweetener, curry powder, cumin, coriander, and red pepper flakes. Sprinkle over the chicken mixture. Top with the sliced basil leaves.

• Cook, covered, on low heat for 8 hours or high heat for 4 hours.

• About 30 minutes before the chicken is done cooking, add the broccoli to the slow cooker.

• When the chicken is almost done cooking, working in batches, in a food processor or blender, gently pulse the cauliflower just until it becomes the texture of rice.

• Lightly coat a large skillet with cooking spray. Cook the cauliflower, salt, and pepper over medium heat for 5 minutes, or until the cauliflower is tender, stirring occasionally.

• Put the cauliflower rice into serving bowls. Sprinkle with the parsley.

• Serve the curry over the rice. Top with the garnishes.

Avocado and Shrimp Spring Rolls

1. Calories 170 Per Serving
2. Protein 7g Per Serving
3. Fiber 9g Per Serving

Ingredients

Servings: 6

Serving Size   2 rolls

• 1 ounce dried rice noodles

• 1 tablespoon peanut sauce

• 4 12-inch Vietnamese salad roll wrappers

• 3 ounces cooked, peeled, and deveined shrimp, tails discarded, halved crosswise

• 1 medium avocado, halved and cut into 12 slices

• 1 medium mango, peeled and cut into julienne strips

• 1 cup tightly packed red leaf lettuce, torn into bite-size pieces

• 1/4 cup tightly packed fresh basil (Thai preferred), stems discarded, torn into bite-size pieces

• 1/4 cup tightly packed fresh mint, stems discarded, torn into bite-size pieces

• 1 2.5-ounce package radish sprouts, steamed (optional)

Directions

• Put 2 cups of water in a small saucepan. Boil over high heat.

• Put the rice noodles in a small, heat-resistant bowl. Pour the boiling water over the noodles. Let stand for 4 minutes, or until the noodles have softened. Drain well in a fine-mesh sieve. Transfer back to the bowl. Stir in the peanut sauce. Set aside.

• Fill a large bowl with warm water. Working with one wrapper at a time, soak the wrapper in the water for 30 seconds, or until just pliable but not limp. Transfer the wrapper to a wooden cutting board. On the wrapper, layer one fourth of each down the center as follows: the shrimp, avocado, mango, lettuce, basil, mint, and sprouts. Top with the rice noodles. Fold the bottom of the wrapper over the filling. Fold in the ends, rolling like a burrito into a tight cylinder. Repeat with the remaining wrappers and ingredients. Transfer the rolls with the seam side down to a plate. Cover with a damp kitchen towel and refrigerate.

• When ready to serve, using a wet knife, cut each roll into thirds. Transfer to a serving platter.

Quick Tips

1. Tip: Wood surfaces are best when working with salad roll wrappers. They tend to stick to plastic cutting boards.

2. Keep it Healthy: The Centers for Disease Control and Prevention (CDC) and the Food and Drug Administration (FDA) don't recommend eating raw sprouts due to potential foodborne illnesses. Before eating sprouts of any kind, be sure to cook them thoroughly, such as steaming them in a steamer basket for 5 minutes, to kill any harmful bacteria.

Chicken Shawarma

1. Calories 202 Per Serving

2. Protein 27g Per Serving

3. Fiber 3g Per Serving

Ingredients

Servings: 4

Serving Size: 3 ounces chicken, 3/4 cup vegetables, and 1 1/2 teaspoons feta

• 2 teaspoons olive oil

• 1 small onion, chopped

• 1 pound boneless, skinless chicken breasts, all visible fat discarded, cut into 1/2 x 2-inch strips

• 1/2 cup fat-free, low-sodium chicken broth

• 4 medium garlic cloves, minced

• 1 teaspoon ground cumin

• 1 teaspoon paprika

• 1/2 teaspoon ground turmeric

• 1/2 teaspoon pepper (coarsely ground preferred)

• 1/4 teaspoon salt

• 2 cups torn romaine lettuce

• 1 medium tomato, sliced, and 1 medium tomato, chopped, divided use

• 1/2 medium unpeeled cucumber, sliced, and 1/2 medium unpeeled cucumber, chopped, divided use

• 2 tablespoons crumbled low-fat feta cheese

• 2 tablespoons minced fresh Italian (flat-leaf) parsley

Directions

• Heat the oil in the pressure cooker on sauté. Cook the onion for 3 minutes, or until soft, stirring frequently. Add the chicken. Cook the chicken for 4 to 6 minutes, or until lightly browned, stirring frequently. Turn off the pressure cooker.

• Stir in the broth, garlic, cumin, paprika, turmeric, pepper, and salt. Secure the lid. Cook on high pressure for 4 minutes. Quickly release the pressure.

• Arrange as follows on a platter: the romaine, sliced tomato, and sliced cucumber. Using a slotted spoon, place the chicken on the cucumbers. Top with the remaining chopped cucumber and chopped tomato. Sprinkle with the feta and parsley.

Simple Persian Salad

1. Calories 88 Per Serving
2. Protein 3g Per Serving

3. Fiber 3g Per Serving

Ingredients

Servings: 4

• 2 medium cucumbers, unpeeled, seeded, and diced

• 4 medium tomatoes, seeded and diced

• 1 medium red onion, diced

• 2 tablespoons fat-free feta cheese, crumbled

• 1/4 cup chopped fresh mint or parsleyOR

• 1 tablespoon plus 1 teaspoon dried mint or parsley, crumbled

• Juice of 2 medium limes

• 1 tablespoon extra-virgin olive oil

• 1/2 teaspoon pepper

Directions

• In a small bowl, stir together the cucumber, tomatoes, onion, feta, and mint. Refrigerate, covered, for 20 minutes.

• In a small bowl, whisk together the lime juice, oil and pepper.

• Pour over the cucumber mixture, tossing to coat.

Veggie Tacos

1. Calories 310 Per Servin

2. Protein 13g Per Serving

3. Fiber 7g Per Serving

Ingredients

Servings: 4

Serving Size: 2 tacos

• 2 tablespoons vegetable oil

• 1 white onion (thinly sliced)

• 1 cup sliced mushrooms

• 8 white corn tortillas

• optional salt

• 1 avocado (thinly sliced)

• 1 deseeded poblano pepper (cut into thin strips)

• 1 cup fat-free feta cheese

Directions

• In a frying pan add the oil and once hot, add onion, poblano peppers, and mushrooms and let brown over low heat. Add a little water to avoid burning.

• Once the vegetables are tender, add fat free feta cheese and season with a little salt (optional).

• Warm tortillas.

• To assemble tacos: First place a slice of avocado on the warmed tortilla followed by a little of the prepared mixture.

Whole Wheat Spaghetti with Marinara and Turkey Meatballs

1. Calories 489 Per Serving

2. Protein 36g Per Serving

3. Fiber 16g Per Serving

Ingredients

Servings 6

Marinara Sauce

• 14 oz. canned, no-salt-added, or, low-sodium, sliced carrots

• 14.4 oz. packaged, frozen pepper stir-fry (onions and peppers) (thawed)

• 1 medium zucchini (chopped)

• 4 clove fresh garlic (minced)OR

• 2 tsp. jarred, minced garlic

• 52 oz. cubed, no-salt-added, or, low-sodium tomato (crushed)

• 2 tsp. salt-free, dried Italian spice blend

Whole Wheat Spaghetti and Turkey Meatballs

• 1 lb. extra-lean or fat-free ground turkey breast (95%-99% lean)

• 1/4 tsp. black pepper

• 1/2 cup whole-grain cereal flakes (crushed, optional)

• 1 lb. whole-wheat spaghetti

Directions

Marinara Sauce

• In a large pot (not over any heat yet), add carrots. Use a fork or potato masher to mash. Add stir-fry vegetables, zucchini, garlic, crushed tomatoes, and spice blend.

• Bring to a boil over high heat. Cover, and reduce heat to medium-low so sauce is simmering.

Whole Wheat Spaghetti and Turkey Meatballs

• In a bowl, combine turkey, pepper, cereal and parsley. Form meat mixture into golf-size meatballs to make about 20 to 25 meatballs.

• Add meatballs into the simmering sauce, trying to get the majority of meatballs covered by sauce. Cover and cook until meatballs are cooked through, about 20 to 25 minutes.

• Make spaghetti according to package directions (omitting the salt and fat). Serve with marinara and meatballs.

Quick Tips

1. Cooking Tip: There are several kid-friendly kid steps in this recipe. Kids can help mash the carrots, crush the cereal in a sealed plastic bag, and use clean hands to form the meatballs.

2. Keep it Healthy: Make sure to compare sodium levels in several brands of canned vegetables and choose the product with the least amount of sodium you can find in your store.

3. Tip: Products simply labeled "ground turkey" will likely also include the skin, which elevates fat and calorie levels greatly. Make sure to purchase "ground turkey breast" which includes only the lean breast meat.

Hearty and Heart-Healthy Potato Soup

1. Calories 131 Per Serving

2. Protein 8g Per Serving

3. Fiber 4g Per Serving

Ingredients

Servings: 8

Serving Size: 1 C

• 2 pounds potatoes, scrubbed and cut in 1/2-inch cubes (about 5 cups)

• 1 tablespoon olive oil

• 2 10-ounce packages frozen chopped onions

• 1/4 cup chopped, dried tomatoes

• 2 pints plus 1 14-ounce can (46 ounces total) low-sodium chicken broth

• 2 cups shredded, cooked turkey

• 3 cups packaged, chopped, frozen mixed vegetables, thawed

• freshly-ground black pepper

Directions

• In heavy soup pot, heat oil on high and stir in onions. Cook, stirring occasionally for about 20 minutes or until well browned.

• Add potatoes, dried tomatoes and broth.

• Bring to boil and cook covered for 10 minutes or until tender.

• Add turkey and vegetables, return to boil and cook 6 - 8 minutes.

• Top with freshly ground pepper.

Hummus

1. Calories 126 Per Serving
2. Protein 6g Per Serving
3. Fiber 4g Per Serving

Ingredients

Servings 8

• 30 ounces canned, low-sodium garbanzo beans (chickpeas) (drained, rinsed)

• 1/2 cup lemon juice

- 2 tsp. minced garlic (from jar)

- 1 Tbsp. extra virgin olive oil

- 1/4 tsp. paprika

- 1/2 tsp. dried parsley

Directions

• Place all ingredients in a blender or food processor and blend until smooth.

• Serve with veggie slices or sticks as a dip.

Avocado, Banana, Orange and Yogurt Smoothie

1. Calories 170 Per Serving
2. Protein 4g Per Serving
3. Fiber 4g Per Serving

Ingredients

Servings: 4

Serving Size: 1/4 recipe

- 1 avocado (halved, pitted, peeled)

• 1/2 banana

• 1 1/2 cups orange juice

• 6 ounces low-fat vanilla yogurt

• 1 cup ice

Directions

• In blender, combine all ingredients until smooth.

Mediterranean Salad

1. Calories 142 Per Serving
2. Protein 8g Per Serving
3. Fiber 4g Per Serving
4. Cost Per Serving

Ingredients

Servings 4

• 1 medium head lettuce (green leaf, red leaf or romaine), cut into thin strips

• 1 medium cucumber, chopped

• 1/2 cup tomatoes, chopped

• 1 15.5-ounce can no-salt-added chickpeas, rinsed and drained

• 1/2 medium red onion, finely sliced

• 1/2 cup crumbled fat-free or low-fat feta cheeseOR

• 1/2 cup shredded Parmesan cheese

• 2 tablespoons extra-virgin olive oil

• 2 tablespoons red wine vinegarOR

• 2 tablespoons cider vinegar

• 1/2 teaspoon garlic powder

• 1/2 teaspoon pepper

Directions

• In a large bowl, gently toss the lettuce, cucumber, tomatoes, chickpeas, onion, and feta.

• In a small bowl, whisk together the oil, vinegar, garlic powder, and pepper.

• Pour the dressing over the salad, tossing to combine.

Black Beans and Rice

1. Calories 363 Per Serving

2. Protein 10g Per Serving

3. Fiber 7g Per Serving

Ingredients

Servings: 4

Serving Size: 1 1/2 cups

• 2 cups uncooked instant brown rice

• ¼ cup fresh lime juice (about 2 medium limes)

• 2 teaspoons olive oil (extra-virgin preferred) and 2 tablespoons olive oil (extra-virgin preferred), divided use

• 1/2 teaspoon salt

• 1 medium onion, finely chopped

• 2 medium garlic cloves, mincedOR

• 1 teaspoon jarred minced garlic

• 2 teaspoons ground cumin

• 1 teaspoon chili powder

• 1 15-ounce can no-salt-added black beans, rinsed and drained

• 2 tablespoons finely chopped fresh cilantro (optional)

• 2 tablespoons finely chopped fresh oregano (optional)

Directions

• Prepare the rice using the package directions, omitting the salt and margarine.

• Meanwhile, in a small bowl, whisk together the lime juice, 2 teaspoons oil and salt. Set aside.

• Heat the remaining 2 tablespoons oil in a large skillet over medium-high heat, swirling to coat the bottom. Cook the onion for 3 minutes, or until soft, stirring frequently. Stir in the garlic. Cook for 1 minute, stirring frequently. Stir in the cumin and chili powder. Cook for 1 minute, stirring frequently. Stir in the beans. Cook until warmed through. Remove from the heat. Transfer to a large serving bowl.

• Stir in the cooked rice, lime juice mixture, cilantro and oregano.

Ground Beef and Pasta Skillet Primavera

1. Calories 296 Per Serving

2. Protein 32g Per Serving

3. Fiber 3g Per Serving

Ingredients

Servings: 4

Serving Size:1 1/2 cup beef and pasta mixture

• 1 pound 96% lean ground beef

• 1 (14-1/2 ounces) can reduced-sodium beef broth

• 1 cup uncooked, whole-wheat pasta

• 2 zucchini or yellow squash, cut in half lengthwise, then crosswise into 1/2-inch slice

• 1 can (14-1/2 ounces) no-salt added diced tomatoes

• 1 1/2 teaspoons Italian seasoning

Directions

• Heat large nonstick skillet over medium heat until hot. Add Ground Beef; cook 8 to 10 minutes, breaking into 3/4-inch crumbles and stirring occasionally. Pour off drippings.

• Stir in broth, pasta, squash, tomatoes and Italian seasoning; bring to a boil. Reduce heat, cover and cook 9 to

11 minutes or until pasta and squash are almost tender and sauce is slightly thickened, stirring occasionally.

Heart-Healthy Nicoise Salad

1. Calories 177 Per Serving

2. Protein 12g Per Serving

3. Fiber 3g Per Serving

Ingredients

Servings: 6

Serving Size approx. 2 C

• 1 1/2 - 2 pounds potatoes, peeled (if desired) and cut into 1/2-inch cubes; approx. 4-5 cup

• 1/2 cup bottled, reduced-calorie ranch salad dressing

• 1-2 teaspoons curry powder (to taste)

• 2 6-ounce cans tuna (packed in water), drained

• 1 cup green onions (chopped)

• 1/2 cup pitted olives (black or green), chopped

• 4 - 6 cups washed and drained mixed salad greens

• 6 plum tomatoes, quartered lengthwise

• 4 hard boiled egg whites, quartered lengthwise

Directions

• Over high heat, bring a large pot of water to boil. Add cubed potatoes; return to boiling and simmer 5 minutes or until tender, but firm. Drain potatoes and set aside or refrigerate.

• In a large bowl, mix together ranch dressing and curry powder to taste. Stir in tuna, green onions and olives. Gently stir in potatoes.

• To serve, arrange greens on a platter (or on individual dishes), top with potato mixture, then garnish with tomatoes and eggs.

Shrimp Ceviche

1. Calories 134 Per Serving
2. Protein 15g Per Serving
3. Fiber 3g Per Serving

Ingredients

Servings 8

• 1 garlic clove

• 1 jalapeño pepper

• 1/2 cup lime juice (fresh)

• 2 Roma tomato

• 1 small red onion

• 1 avocado

• 1/2 bunch fresh cilantro

• 1 pound shrimp (peeled, steamed)

• 1 mango (peeled)

• black pepper (to taste)

Directions

• Using the food processor, chop the garlic clove, jalapeño, Roma tomatoes, and red onion. You can add the lime juice if you need a little liquid to allow the processor to do its job. Place in a large mixing bowl.

• With a knife chop the cilantro, shrimp, mango, and avocado and add it to the mixing bowl. (Do not put these items in food processor, please chop by hand)

• Mix all the ingredients together (including any of the lime juice you didn't already add). Add the black pepper to taste.

Chicken Paella

1. Calories 380 Per Serving

2. Protein 24g Per Serving

3. Fiber 7g Per Serving

4. Cost Per Serving

Ingredients

Servings 6

• Cooking spray

• 1 pound boneless, skinless chicken breasts or tenderloins (all visible fat discarded, cut into 1-inch cubes)

• 2 tsp extra virgin olive oil or vegetable oil

• 1 medium green bell pepper (thinly sliced)

• 1 medium red bell pepper (thinly sliced)

• 1 small onion (chopped)

• 2 medium chopped tomatoes, lightly mashed in a bowl with a fork (save the juices!)

• 1 can no-salt-added green peas

• 1 teaspoon garlic (minced, from jar)

• 1/2 teaspoon parsley

• 1/4 teaspoon saffronOR

- 1/8 teaspoon turmeric
- 1 cup low-sodium chicken or vegetable broth
- 2 cup long-grain rice (cooked to package instructions)

Directions

- Spray a large skillet with cooking spray, add chicken and cook over medium-high heat 5-7 minutes, stirring occasionally.
- Remove chicken from pan.
- Add oil, bell peppers and onions to skillet – stir well and cook 5 minutes until onions begin to become translucent.
- Add tomatoes, peas, garlic, parsley and saffron or Turmeric. Stir and cook 2 minutes more.
- Reduce to medium low-heat, add broth and chicken, stir well and cover.
- Simmer for 20 minutes.
- Add rice, mix well and heat until warmed through.

Curried Cauliflower with Chickpeas

1. Calories 224 Per Serving

2. Protein 11g Per Serving

3. Fiber 11g Per Serving

Ingredients

Servings:4

Serving Size: 1 1/2 C

• 3 cups water

• 3/4 cup dried chickpeas, sorted for stones and shriveled peas, rinsed, and drained

• 2 teaspoons canola or corn oil

• 1 medium onion (chopped)

• 1 medium red bell pepper (chopped)

• 2 tablespoons minced, peeled gingerroot

• 3 medium garlic cloves (minced)

• 1 1/2 cups fat-free, low-sodium vegetable broth

• 1 medium head of cauliflower, cut into bite-size florets

• 2 tablespoons curry powder

• 1/4 teaspoon salt

• 2 tablespoons minced, fresh cilantro (optional)

Directions

• In the pressure cooker, stir together the water and chickpeas. Secure the lid. Cook on high pressure for 45 minutes. Release the pressure naturally for 15 minutes, then quickly release the remaining pressure. Drain the chickpeas in a colander.

• Heat the oil in the pressure cooker on sauté. Cook the onion for 3 minutes, or until soft, stirring frequently. Add the bell pepper. Cook for 3 minutes, or until tender. Stir in the gingerroot and garlic. Cook for 30 seconds, stirring frequently. Turn off the pressure cooker.

• Stir in the broth, cauliflower, curry powder, and salt. Stir in the chickpeas. Secure the lid. Cook on high pressure for 3 minutes. Quickly release the pressure.

• Serve sprinkled with the cilantro.

Cooking Tip:

1. Curry powder is an integral part of this dish and the actual flavor and heat level vary with the brand. If the brand you're using is labeled "Madras," it's hotter than regular curry powder.

2. Once you make this dish, you'll know if you prefer to increase or decrease the amount of curry powder.

Garden Vegetable Stir-Fried Sorghum

1. Calories 282 Per Serving
2. Protein 12g Per Serving
3. Fiber 7g Per Serving

Ingredients

Servings: 4

Serving Size: 1 1/2 cups

- 1 cup uncooked whole grain sorghum
- 2 teaspoons sesame oil
- 2 medium garlic cloves, mincedOR
- 2 teaspoons jarred minced garlic
- 1 teaspoon gingerroot, peeled and minced
- 1 cup broccoli florets, chopped, thawed if frozen
- 1 cup snow peas, trimmed and halved
- 1/2 cup carrot strips, sliced into matchstick-size

• 1/2 cup red bell pepper, diced

• 1/2 cup mushrooms, thinly sliced

• 1/2 cup frozen shelled edamame, thawed

• 2 large eggs

• 1 tablespoon soy sauce (lowest sodium available) and 1 tablespoon soy sauce (lowest sodium available), divided use

• 1/2 cup water chestnuts, rinsed and drained

• 1/4 cup green onions (about 2 medium), green parts only, diagonally sliced

Directions

• Prepare the sorghum using the package directions, omitting the salt. Once cooked, spread the sorghum in an even layer on a rimmed baking sheet or in a 13 x 9 x 2-inch baking dish. Let stand for 5 to 10 minutes at room temperature. Refrigerate, uncovered, for 20 minutes, or until cool.

• In a large nonstick skillet, Dutch oven or wok, heat the oil over medium heat, swirling to coat the bottom. Cook the garlic and gingerroot for 30 seconds, stirring frequently. Increase the heat to medium high. Cook the broccoli, snow peas, carrots, bell pepper, mushrooms and edamame, for 10 to 12 minutes, or until the vegetables are tender-crisp, stirring frequently.

• Meanwhile, in a small bowl, using a fork, beat together the eggs and 1 tablespoon soy sauce.

• Reduce the heat to medium. Stir the water chestnuts and sorghum into the vegetable mixture. Push the mixture to the sides of the skillet. Pour the egg mixture into the center of the skillet. Using a heatproof rubber scraper, stir for 1 to 2 minutes, or until partially set.

• Stir the vegetable mixture into the partially cooked egg mixture. Cook for 1 minute, or until the eggs are cooked through and the sorghum is heated through, stirring constantly. (The USDA recommends cooking egg dishes to 160°F.)

• Remove from the heat. Stir in the remaining 1 tablespoon soy sauce. Sprinkle with the green onions.

Quick Tips

1. Cooking Tip: Why use cold sorghum? The coolness helps to dry out the grains for a better texture. If you start with warm, just-cooked sorghum, your dish will turn out

soggy. To get a jumpstart on the next day's dinner, prepare the sorghum ahead of time and refrigerate, covered, for up to two days.

2. Tip: To save some time, buy the packaged shredded carrots. They're already peeled and cut into thin strips.

Korean Vegetable Pancakes

1. Calories 183 Per Serving
2. Protein 9.0g Per Serving
3. Fiber 5.4g Per Serving

Ingredients

Servings: 4

Serving Size: 2

• 2 1/2 cups ice-cold water

• 1/2 cup roughly chopped carrots

• 1/2 cup roughly chopped zucchini

• 1/2 cup roughly chopped cauliflower

• 1/2 cup roughly chopped broccoli

• 1/4 cup roughly chopped scallions

- 1 1/4 cup all-purpose, whole-wheat flour

- 2 large eggs

- 1/4 teaspoon salt

- 1/4 teaspoon ground black pepper

Directions

- Add enough ice cubes into 2 1/2 cups water to make water ice-cold.

- In the bowl of a food processor, add carrots, zucchini, cauliflower, broccoli, and scallions. Pulse to puree vegetables until finely chopped-but be careful not to turn the vegetables into liquid.

- Into a large bowl, add flour, eggs, salt, and pepper. Pour in 2 cups of cold water (without ice cubes). Use a fork to whisk mixture together until combined. Stir in the pureed vegetables. Aim for a pancake-like batter consistency, adding 1 to 2 tablespoons more water if needed.

- Coat an 8-inch nonstick pan with cooking spray and warm over medium-high heat. Add 1/2 cup batter into the center of the pan. Cook until edges begin to get golden-about 2 to 3 minutes-and then use a spatula to carefully flip. Cook another 1 to 2 minutes until the side is golden. Transfer pancake to a plate. Spray pan with cooking spray and repeat continually until all 8 pancakes are made.

Quick Tips

1. Cooking Tip: 2 cups of any finely chopped vegetables can be used in this recipe, not just the ones listed—anything from green beans to peas to bell peppers to cabbage. Just purée in the food processor like instructed in recipe.

2. Keep it Healthy: Pancakes aren't just for breakfast. Smear a little fat-free cream cheese onto half the pancake, fold into quarters or roll up, and pack into a school lunchbox for a different sort of sandwich for your children.

3. Tip: To make a dipping sauce for the pancakes, mix together 2 tablespoons less-sodium soy sauce, 1 tablespoon water, and 1 tablespoon white vinegar together with 1/2 teaspoon granulated sugar and 1/2 teaspoon (optional) hot red pepper flakes.

Creole Steak with Jambalaya Rice

1. Calories 338 Per Serving
2. Protein 29g Per Serving
3. Fiber 4.7g Per Serving

Ingredients

Servings: 4

Serving Size: 1/4 cup rice mix, 1/2 cup sliced steak

• 1 1/2 cups cooked brown rice

• 1 cup chopped celery

• 2 1/2 teaspoons Creole seasoning, divided

• 1 cup chopped green bell pepper

• 1 cup chopped onion

• 1 lb sirloin tip steaks, cut-1/4 inch thick

• 1 can (14 1/2 ounces) no salt added diced tomatoes

• 2 tablespoons vegetable oil (divided)

Directions

• Heat 1 tablespoon oil over medium heat in 3-quart saucepan until hot. Add onion, celery, bell pepper and 1 teaspoon Creole seasoning; cook 8 to 10 minutes or until vegetables are crisp-tender, stirring occasionally.

• Stir in tomatoes and rice. Cover and continue cooking 2 to 4 minutes or until heated through, stirring occasionally. Keep warm.

• Meanwhile, press remaining 1-1/2 teaspoons Creole seasoning evenly onto beef steaks. Heat 1-1/2 teaspoons oil in large nonstick skillet over medium-high heat until hot. Cooking in batches, place steaks in skillet (do not overcrowd) and cook 1 to 3 minutes for medium rare (145°F) doneness, turning once. (Do not overcook.) Remove from skillet; keep warm. Repeat with remaining steaks and oil.

• Serve steaks topped with rice mixture.

Sweet and Spicy Edamame

1. Calories 136 Per Serving

2. Protein 11g Per Serving

3. Fiber 4g Per Serving

Ingredients

Servings: 4

Serving Size: 1/2 cup

• 2 cups water

• 1/2 teaspoon stevia sweetenerOR

• 1 stevia sweetener packet

• 10 drops clear-flavored liquid stevia sweetener

• 2 cups frozen, shelled edamame (green soybeans)OR

• 4 1/2 cups frozen edamame pods

• 1 tablespoon soy sauce (lowest sodium available)

• 2 teaspoons Sriracha hot sauce

• 1 teaspoon toasted sesame oil

• 1 teaspoon grated, peeled gingerroot

• 1 medium garlic clove (minced)

• 1/8 teaspoon black pepper

• 1 tablespoon plus 1 teaspoon sesame seeds

• 1 tablespoon plain rice vinegar

Directions

• Put the water, stevia sweetener, and liquid stevia sweetener in a medium saucepan. Stir together. Bring to a boil over high heat, stirring occasionally. Stir in the edamame. Cook for 3 to 5 minutes, or until tender, stirring occasionally. Drain the edamame in a colander, discarding the water mixture. Set aside.

• In the same saucepan, heat the soy sauce, rice vinegar, Sriracha, sesame oil, gingerroot, garlic, and pepper over low heat for 1 to 2 minutes, stirring occasionally. Add the edamame, tossing to coat.

• Sprinkle the sesame seeds over the edamame.

Quick Tips

1. To eat edamame that's still in the pod, bring the pod to your lips, then squeeze or bite the beans into your mouth. You don't eat the pod, just the edamame beans inside, which will easily pop out.

Moroccan Lentil Stew with Butternut Squash

1. Calories 270 Per Serving

2. Protein 17g Per Serving

3. Fiber 10g Per Serving

Ingredients

Servings: 8

Serving Size: 1 1/2 cups

• 1 teaspoon canola oilOR

• 1 teaspoon corn oil

• 1 medium onion (yellow preferred), diced

• 2 medium garlic cloves or 1 teaspoon jarred minced garlic (optional)

• 1 1/2 teaspoons ground cumin

• 1 1/2 teaspoons ground coriander

• 1 teaspoon ground cinnamon

• 1/2 teaspoon salt

• 1/4 teaspoon pepper

• 1 2-pound butternut squash, peeled, seeds and strings discarded, and chopped into 1-inch cubes (about 4 cups)OR

• 20 ounces frozen butternut squash cubes

• 5 cups low-sodium vegetable broth

• 1 28-ounce can no-salt-added diced tomatoes

• 1 15-ounce can no-salt-added lentilsOR

• 3/4 cup dried lentils, sorted for stones and shriveled lentils, rinsed, and drained

• 3/4 cup chopped fresh cilantro

• 1 teaspoon grated lemon zest

Directions

• In a large pot or Dutch oven, heat the oil over medium-high heat, swirling to coat the bottom. Cook the onion for 3 minutes, or until soft, stirring frequently.

• Stir in the garlic, cumin, coriander, cinnamon, salt, and pepper. Cook for 1 minute, or until the garlic and spices are fragrant. Stir in the butternut squash, broth, tomatoes, and lentils.

• Bring to a boil. Reduce the heat to low. Simmer, covered, for 40 minutes, or until the lentils are tender. Sprinkle with the cilantro and lemon zest.

Quick Tips

1. Cooking Tip: Ground cinnamon isn't just for desserts. Consider adding it to stews and chilis for a touch of earthiness.

2. Keep it Healthy: If you can't find no-salt-added canned lentils, opt for the dried version.

3. Tip: You can substitute cubed acorn squash or sweet potatoes for the butternut squash.

Blue Smoothie

1. Calories 179 Per Serving

2. Protein 7g Per Serving

3. Fiber 7g Per Serving

Ingredients

Servings: 2

Serving Size: 1½ cups

• 2 cups frozen unsweetened peach slices

• 2 cups tightly packed fresh spinach

• 1 cup frozen unsweetened blueberries

• 1 cup fat-free milk

• 1 teaspoon honey

Directions

• In a food processor or blender, process all the ingredients until smooth, about 1 to 2 minutes, stopping to scrape down the mixture if necessary.

• Pour into glasses.

Quick Tips

1. Cooking Tip: You can substitute ½ cup frozen spinach for the fresh spinach. Just add a few more splashes of milk if necessary.

2. Tip: Using frozen fruit eliminates the need for ice in a smoothie. You can easily use fresh fruit, however, by using the same quantities of fruit and adding 1½ cups of ice cubes.

Sweet Potato and Ricotta Latkes

1. Calories 148 Per Serving
2. Protein 3g Per Serving
3. Fiber 1g Per Serving

Ingredients

Servings: 8

Serving Size:1 pancake

- 12 ounces potatoes, peeled, approx. 2 cups
- 3 tablespoons part-skim ricotta cheese
- 2 tablespoons flour

• 2 tablespoons sugar

• 2 teaspoons finely grated orange zest

• 1 teaspoon baking powder

• 1/4 teaspoon salt

• 1 egg (lightly beaten)

• 1/3 cup raisins

• 1/4 cup vegetable oil

• 4 teaspoons confectioner's sugar

Directions

• Preheat oven to 350° F. Grate potatoes into a large mixing bowl. Stir in ricotta, flour, sugar, orange peel, baking powder and salt. Add eggs and raisins; mix until well combined.

• In a large, heavy, non-stick skillet, heat 1 tablespoon oil over medium heat. Using a tablespoon, spoon potato mixture into skillet, using about 2 tablespoons per pancake. (Skillet should hold about 4 pancakes at a time.) Flatten mixture slightly with a spatula. Cook pancakes 2 minutes, then flip and cook another 2 minutes or until golden brown. Transfer pancakes to a baking sheet while cooking the remaining pancakes.

• Place cooked pancakes in the oven and bake 10 minutes or until pancakes are cooked through.

Cozy Beef Stew

1. Calories 326 Per Serving

2. Protein 35g Per Serving

3. Fiber 8g Per Serving

Ingredients

Servings12

• 4 pounds boneless sirloin steak, all visible fat discarded, cut into 1-inch cubes

• 4 cups baby red potatoes, halved

• 4 cups baby carrots

• 2 medium onions, chopped

• 2 cups chopped celery

• 1 15-ounce can no-salt-added tomato sauce

• 10 ounces dried lima beans, sorted for stones and shriveled beans, rinsed, and drainedOR

• 10 ounces dried black-eyed peas, sorted for stones and shriveled peas, rinsed, and drained

• 2 tablespoons brown sugar

• 1 tablespoon plus 1 teaspoon quick-cooking tapioca

• 2 teaspoons pepper

• 1 teaspoon celery salt

• 1 teaspoon dried parsley, crumbled

• 1 teaspoon dried thyme, crumbled

• 1 cup water

Directions

Directions for Cooking

• If frozen, thaw the bags in the refrigerator overnight. Pour the contents into a slow cooker. Stir in the water. Cook, covered, on low for 4 to 6 hours, or until the vegetables are tender.

Directions for Freezing

• In a large bowl, stir together all the ingredients except the water. Transfer the mixture equally between two 1-gallon resealable plastic freezer bags. Lay the bags flat in the freezer.

Quick Tips

1. Cooking Tip: Don't have celery salt? No problem. Here are a couple substitutions. Using a mortar and pestle or spice grinder, grind enough celery seeds to make 1/2 teapoon ground celery. In a small bowl, stir together the ground celery with 1/4 to 1/2 teaspoon salt. You can also use 1 teaspoon dill salt in place of 1 teaspoon celery salt.

Simple Chicken (or Shrimp) Stir-Fry

1. Calories 349 Per Serving
2. Protein 25g Per Serving
3. Fiber 8g Per Serving

Ingredients

Servings: 4

• Cooking spray

• 1 pound boneless, skinless chicken breast halves, all visible fat discarded, cut into bite-size piecesOR

• 18 raw medium shrimp, peeled, rinsed, and patted dry

• 2 teaspoons canola or corn oilOR

• 2 teaspoons extra-virgin olive oil

• 1/2 medium head green cabbage, thinly sliced

• 4 medium carrots, shredded

• 2 tablespoons soy sauce (lowest sodium available)

• 1 tablespoon low-sodium peanut butter

• 1/2 teaspoon fresh gingerrot, grated (optional)

• 2 cups cooked brown rice, covered to keep warm

• 2 tablespoons chopped unsalted peanuts

Directions

• Lightly spray a large skillet or wok with cooking spray. Cook the chicken over medium-high heat for 5 minutes, or until no longer pink in the center, stirring occasionally. (If using shrimp, cook over medium heat for 3 minutes, or until pink on the outside, stirring frequently.) Transfer to a plate. Set aside.

• In the same skillet, heat the oil over medium-high heat, swirling to coat the bottom. Cook the cabbage and carrots for 4 minutes, or until the carrots are tender-crisp, stirring frequently. Stir in the chicken.

• In a small bowl, whisk together the soy sauce, peanut butter, and gingerroot. Stir into the chicken mixture. Cook for 2 minutes, or until heated through.

• Spoon the rice onto plates. Top with the chicken mixture. Sprinkle with the peanuts.

Quick Tips

1. Tip: You can substitute tofu for the chicken to make this a vegetarian meal. Cut 1 pound low-fat, extra-firm tofu (drained well) into 1/2-inch cubes. When the carrots are tender-crisp, stir in the tofu.

2. Tip: To save time, buy preshredded cabbage and carrots. Prepared and packaged produce can be more convenient, but it is usually more costly, too.

The Ultimate Stroke Diet Smoothie Recipes

PURSLANE-BLUEBERRY SUPERFOOD SMOOTHIE

Yield: 4

Prep time: 5 MINUTES

Total time: 5 MINUTES

INGREDIENTS

- 1 bunch purslane, rinsed
- 8 oz frozen blueberries
- 1/2 cup plain yogurt
- 1/4 cup filtered water (add more as needed)

INSTRUCTIONS

1. Whether you procured your yard, your CSA, the farmers market or a nursery, it's likely going to need a good rinse to remove dirt, etc.

2. Once rinsed, place the purslane, blueberries, banana, yogurt and water into a Vitamix or blender and blend until smooth. Add additional water as needed to reach your favorite consistency.

3. Give it a taste. Need a little extra sweetness? Add some honey, agave or deseeded dates. Blend again. And, enjoy!

Cholesterol-Lowering Spinach Mango Smoothie Recipe

PREP TIME: 2 minutes
COOK TIME: 1 minute
TOTAL TIME: 1 minute

Ingredients

- 1/2 avocado

- 1 cup mango, frozen, chunks

- 1 cup spinach

- 1 cup coconut water, unsweetened

- 1 tablespoon chia seeds

- 1 cup ice

• 1 scoop Collagen Boost, optional

Instructions

1. Place avocado, mango, spinach, coconut water, chia seeds, and ice into a blender and secure the lid.

2. Start the blender on its lowest speed and steadily ramp up to its highest speed. This will reduce wear and tear on the motor and blades, facilitate a more consistent blend, and help prevent food splatter onto the lid and sides.

3. Blend for approximately 30 seconds or until a smooth consistency is achieved.

4. Pour into a glass for immediate refreshment or place in the refrigerator in an airtight container to enjoy later.

Notes

1. If you don't have frozen fruit, or simply prefer to use fresh fruit (we totally get that), we recommend adding 1/2 cup of ice to chill your smoothie and give it a pleasing icy texture.

2. You can substitute kale for spinach or add a scoop of protein powder for an extra protein boost.

3. For a sweeter smoothie, you can add a small amount of honey or a few drops of stevia.

4. If you prefer a creamier texture, you can replace coconut water with almond milk or any other milk of your choice.

Banana Mango Smoothie Recipe

Ingredients

- 1 large banana
- 1 cup of mango
- 1 persimmon
- 4 tbsp. of oatmeal
- 1 tsp. of honey

Instructions

1. Fill the Nutribullet cup, add milk to the max line and blend.

Kiwi Pineapple Spinach Smoothie Recipe

Ingredients

• 1 avocado, peeled and pitted

• 2 kiwi, peeled

• 1 1/2 cups lightly packed fresh baby spinach

• 1 cup frozen pineapple chunks

• 1 banana, peeled

• 1 cup plain low fat greek yogurt

• 1/2 cup milk

Instructions

• Place all the ingredients into the pitcher of a high powered blender.

• Blend the ingredients together until smooth, approximately 1-2 minutes.

• Divide the smoothie between 2 8-ounce glasses or 4 4-ounce glasses and serve immediately.

Notes

1. Smoothie is best served immediately after making it

Chocolate Raspberry Protein Smoothie Recipe

Ingredients

- 1 cup chocolate almond milk

- 2 scoops chocolate protein

- 1 cup fresh raspberries

- 1/4 cup chocolate almond butter

- 1 tablespoon chia seeds

- 1 cup ice cubes

- cocoa powder for garnish

Instructions

1. Combine all ingredients in blender (minus cocoa powder).

2. Blend until smooth.

3. Pour into serving glasses and dust with cocoa powder if desired.

4. Enjoy your Chocolate Raspberry Protein Smoothie Recipe!

Strawberry Smoothie

Ingredients

• Frozen Strawberries half cup

• Yogurt half cup

• Milk Half cup

• 3-4 Tbsp Sugar

Cooking Instructions

• Washed strawberries place in box sprinle sugar to cover all strawberties and freeze them.

• take half cup frozen strawberry add half cup cold yogurt and half cup cold milk sugar is not needed as strawberries are already coated in sugar but if you want it sweeter then add 2 to 4 tbsp sugar also. blend everything until smooth.... you can make mango peach cheeko banana smoothie in same way....

Antioxidant Smoothie

Cook Time

- Preparation: 6 minReady in: 6 min
- For: 4 Servings

Ingredients

- 1 cup fresh or frozen beets
- 1 cup fresh or frozen blueberries
- 1 cup fresh or frozen dragon fruit
- 1 cup fresh or frozen strawberries
- 2 cups pineapple juice

Instructions

1. In a high-speed blender, add beets, blueberries, dragon fruit, strawberries, Add pineapple juice, and process until smooth. Add sweetener to taste and serve immediately.

Dairy-Free Chocolate Peanut Butter Banana Smoothie

SERVES: 1

CUISINE: American

CATEGORY: Smoothies

PREP TIME: 10 mins

TOTAL TIME: 10 mins

INGREDIENTS:

• 1-1/2 cup almond milk

• 1/4 cup crushed ice

• 1 tablespoon ground flaxseed

• 2 tablespoons creamy natural peanut butter (unsweetened)

• 1/2 tablespoon honey (or sweetener of your choice)

• 1/8 teaspoon vanilla extract

• 1 frozen banana (very ripe)

• 1 tablespoon raw cacao powder

INSTRUCTIONS:

1. Blend all of the ingredients in a blender or vitamix! It's as easy as that.

2. Enjoy immediately!

Parsley-Passion Green Smoothie

Category: Drink

Servings: 3

Prep Time: 50 minutes

Calories: 77

Ingredients

- 1 1/2 cups water
- 1/2 cucumber cut lengthwise
- 1 banana
- 1 cup pineapple chunks
- 1/4 bunch of parsley approximately ½ cup
- 1 cup ice cubes

Directions

1. Add ingredients to FourSide or WildSide+ jar in order listed and secure lid.

2. Select "Whole Juice" or blend on a Medium-High speed for 50-60 seconds.

High Potassium Smoothie

PREP TIME: 5 minutes
TOTAL TIME: 5 minutes
SERVINGS: 2
CALORIES: 351 kcal

EQUIPMENT

• 1 Blender

INGREDIENTS

• ½ avocado

• ½ cup mango frozen

• 1 cup spinach frozen

• 1 banana

• 3 tbsp hemp seeds

• 1 cup unsweetened soy milk

INSTRUCTIONS

- In a blender add all the ingredients together

- Bluend until smooth

- Serve cold and enjoy!

Pineapple Green Smoothie

PREP: 5 MINUTES

TOTAL: 5 MINUTES

COURSE: SMOOTHIE

CUISINE: PLANT-BASED

SERVES: 1

EQUIPMENT

- High-speed blender

INGREDIENTS

- 1 cup kale

- 1 cup coconut water unsweetened

- ½ orange peeled

- ¼ cucumber peeled

• 1 cup pineapple frozen

• ¼ lemon peeled

• 1 serving homemade protein powder optional

INSTRUCTIONS

• Blend kale, coconut water, and orange together until smooth.

• Add remaining ingredients and blend again.

NOTES

• Use at least one frozen fruit to make smoothie cold

• Swap coconut water with regular water

• Keep the white pith on the orange and lemon for added nutrition

• Add a plant-based protein powder like my protein powder recipe to help your body process the natural sugars from this smoothie

• Feel free to swap kale for the leafy greens of your choice

Strawberry Beet Smoothie

PREP TIME: 5 minutes

TOTAL TIME: 5minutes

COURSE: Breakfast

INGREDIENTS

- 1 cup Strawberries fresh or frozen

- 1 Beet peeled and chopped

- 1/2 Lemon peeled

- 2 stalks Celery roughly chopped

- 2 tbsp Hemp seeds

- 2 tbsp Chia seeds

- 1 tbsp Almond butter

- 1 cup Water (or you can sub unsweetened almond milk)

INSTRUCTIONS

- Place all ingredients into a high speed blender and blend until smooth. Enjoy!

- If this smoothie is not sweet enough for you, try adding an apple to sweeten it up.

NOTES

1. If you don't have a high-speed blender, you may want to steam your beet first before blending.

Healthy Mango Banana Smoothie

Ingredients

• 1 medium size mango, peeled.

• 1 medium ripe banana.

• 1 cup milk (I used whole milk; you may use almond milk or any nut milk)

• 1 tablespoon coconut flakes.

• 1 tablespoon hemp seeds

• Optional: You may add 1 tablespoon chia seeds and peanut butter or any nut butter

Directions

• Combine all ingredients in a blender and blend on high speed until smooth.

• Pour in a glass, top with any toppings of choice

• Enjoy

Tips

1. You can freeze left over smoothies in ice trays or popsicle mold for those hot summer days.

GREEN CLEANSING SMOOTHIE

TOTAL TIME: 10 minutes

COURSE: Breakfast, Drinks

SERVINGS: 2 people

CALORIES: 116 kcal

EQUIPMENT

• Blender

INGREDIENTS

• 100 ml cold green tea

• 100 ml filter water

• 30 g frozen spinach

• 1 frozen banana

• 2 celery stalks

• 1 tsp manuka honey

- ½ juiced lime

- ½ apple

- ½ kiwi

- ½ tsp spirulina optional

INSTRUCTIONS

• Leave frozen bananas on the side and allow a few minutes to defrost a little bit.

• Place all ingredients into the blender and blend for a minute until smooth.

• Enjoy this 100% healthy drink

NOTES

1. I will be lying if I tell you, this will be the most favorite drink ever. However, bearing in mind all its benefits, it definitely should be included in our weekly meal plans to reach 15 plant based diversity! If you interested to know more about food diversity and how important it's for our wellbeing, keep an eye for new blog post as I'm planning to write an article on this topic.

PINEAPPLE CUCUMBER CREAMY SMOOTHIE RECIPE

SERVING: 1

PREP TIME: 5 minutes

EQUIPMENT

Knife

Cutting board

Measuring cup

High-speed blender ready.

INGREDIENTS

1. 1 whole cucumber

2. 1 small pineapple

3. 1 cup of Real California Milk

4. 1 teaspoon of manuka honey

5. Half a cup of ice cubes

INSTRUCTIONS

1. Measure a cup of Real California Milk into a bowl. Cut the cucumber and pineapple onto a plate. Set aside. P.S.

You don't have to peel off the cucumber skin as it is rich in dietary fiber and nutrients. Just wash thoroughly under running water and cut into slices.

2. Measure the ice cubes or crushed ice into the blender. Then pour the milk in, add the pineapple and cucumber slices, and drizzle in the manuka honey.

3. Blend the ingredients for 15-20 seconds or until the ice is completely crushed and the smoothie is smooth and creamy.

4. Pour your pineapple cucumber creamy smoothie into a glass and enjoy immediately. As much as I enjoyed the sweet tropical flavor of pineapple, refreshing mildly sweet taste of cucumber, and the lingering earthy taste of manuka honey, I have to say that the star ingredient of this smoothie recipe is Real California Milk. It gives the smoothie a luxurious texture, rich sweet taste, and ups its nutritional value by adding much-needed protein and essential vitamins and minerals.

Green Berry Kefir Smoothie

Total Time: 10 minutes

Servings: 1 serving

Ingredients

- 1 cup low fat or nonfat plain kefir
- 1 cup frozen blueberries
- ½ teaspoon chia seeds
- 1 small banana
- 1 teaspoon honey
- ½ cup baby spinach

Instructions

- Place all ingredients in Vitamix/blender and process until smooth.

Avocado, Banana, Orange and Yogurt Smoothie

1. Calories 170 Per Serving

2. Protein 4g Per Serving

3. Fiber 4g Per Serving

Ingredients

Servings: 4

Serving Size: 1/4 recipe

• 1 avocado (halved, pitted, peeled)

• 1/2 banana

• 1 1/2 cups orange juice

• 6 ounces low-fat vanilla yogurt

• 1 cup ice

Directions

• In blender, combine all ingredients until smooth.

Blue Smoothie

1. Calories 179 Per Serving

2. Protein 7g Per Serving

3. Fiber 7g Per Serving

Ingredients

Servings: 2

Serving Size: 1½ cups

• 2 cups frozen unsweetened peach slices

• 2 cups tightly packed fresh spinach

• 1 cup frozen unsweetened blueberries

• 1 cup fat-free milk

• 1 teaspoon honey

Directions

• In a food processor or blender, process all the ingredients until smooth, about 1 to 2 minutes, stopping to scrape down the mixture if necessary.

• Pour into glasses.

Quick Tips

1. Cooking Tip: You can substitute ½ cup frozen spinach for the fresh spinach. Just add a few more splashes of milk if necessary.

2. Tip: Using frozen fruit eliminates the need for ice in a smoothie. You can easily use fresh fruit, however, by using

the same quantities of fruit and adding 1½ cups of ice cubes.

Tropical Green Smoothie

1. Calories 168 Per Serving
2. Protein 3g Per Serving
3. Fiber 6g Per Serving

Ingredients

Servings: 2

• 2 handfuls spinach

• 1 cup coconut water

• 1 tablespoon flax seeds

• 1 teaspoon honey

• 1 medium orange

• 3/4 cup frozen mango chunks

• 1/2 medium banana

• 2 cups ice

Directions

• In a food processor or blender, process the spinach, water, and honey until blended.

• Add the orange, mango, and banana. Process until smooth.

• Add the ice, 1/4 cup at a time, until the desired consistency.

BRAIN POWER SMOOTHIE (BLUEBERRY AVOCADO SMOOTHIE)

• Prep time: 1 MINUTES
• Cook time: 1 MINUTES
• Total time: 2 MINUTES
• Yield: ABOUT 4 CUPS

INGREDIENTS

• 2 cups blueberries
• 1 cup pomegranate juice (or any berry juice)
• 1 cup ice cubes
• 1 Tbsp. chia seeds

• 1 ripe banana, peeled

• half of an avocado, peeled and pitted

INSTRUCTIONS

• Add all ingredients to a blender and pulse until combined and smooth. If the smoothie is too thick, add more juice. If the smoothie is too thin, add more ice.

Triple Berry Protein Smoothie

1. Calories 78 Per Serving

2. Protein 7g Per Serving

3. Fiber 2g Per Serving

Ingredients

Servings: 2

Serving Size: 1 cup

• 1 cup unsweetened almond milk

• 1/2 cup fat-free, plain Greek yogurt

• 1 teaspoon stevia sweetenerOR

• 2 stevia sweetener packets

- 1 squeeze mixed berry-flavored stevia water enhancer

- 1/4 cup fresh or frozen, unsweetened blueberries

- 1/4 cup fresh or frozen, unsweetened raspberries

- 1/4 cup fresh or frozen, unsweetened strawberries

Directions

- In a food processor or blender, process all the ingredients for 1 to 2 minutes, or until the desired texture. Pour into glasses.

Potassium Power Smoothie

Servings: 3 PRINT

Prep Time 5 minutes

Total Time 6 minutes

INGREDIENTS

- 1 ripe, fresh avocado, halved, pitted, and peeled

- 1 ripe banana, peeled and sliced

- 1 kiwi fruit, peeled and sliced

- 1 1/2 cups fortified soy milk (or favorite milk alternative)

- 1 cup ice cubes

DIRECTIONS

1. Place avocado, banana, kiwi, soy milk and ice cubes in a blender. Cover and blend until smooth. Pour into glasses and serve immediately.

Pomegranate Power Smoothie

Yield: 4 servings

Ingredients:

1. 1 cup fat-free milk

2. ½ cup vanilla non-fat Greek yogurt

3. 1 cup frozen peach slices

4. ½ cup frozen dark sweet cherries

5. ½ banana, sliced

6. 1 cup pomegranate juice

7. 3 ice cubes

8. 3 medjool dates, pitted

9. ½ teaspoon Kroger ground cinnamon

10. 1/4 teaspoon Kroger vanilla extract

11. 2 Tablespoons pomegranate seeds (optional)

Directions:

1. Place fat-free milk, yogurt, peach slices, cherries, banana slices, pomegranate juice, ice, dates, ground cinnamon and vanilla extract in blender. Blend on high until smooth. Divide between four glasses and top with pomegranate seeds (optional).

Heart-Healthy Smoothie

PREP TIME: 5 minutes

COOK TIME: 1 minute

SERVINGS: 1

Ingredients

1. 1 cup frozen berries

2. ½ cup raw red beets, peeled and diced small

3. 1 small banana, sliced

4. ½ cup unsweetened almond milk (or preferred milk)

5. 1 tablespoon chia seeds

6. ¼ teaspoon cinnamon

7. pinch fine sea salt

Directions

1. Peel and dice ½ cup raw red beets. Slice 1 small banana.

2. Combine all of your ingredients in a blender, and blend everything until smooth.

3. Enjoy

Green Smoothie

PREP TIME: 5 min
TOTAL TIME: 5 min

Ingredients

1. 2 cups 1 percent milk or nondairy milk of your choice

2. 1 large ripe banana

3. 2 cups fresh baby spinach, packed1 cup frozen mango chunks

4. 2 tbsp ground flaxseeds (optional)

Directions

1. Add all ingredients to a blender and blend until completely smooth, about 1 minute. Stir as needed to allow all ingredients to blend fully.

Strawberry Flax Smoothie Bowl

TOTAL TIME: 5 MIN
PREP TIME: 5 MIN

Ingredients

- ½ frozen banana

- ½ cup frozen strawberries

- ½ cup almond milk or milk of choice, unsweetened

- 2 tablespoons ground flax

- 2 teaspoons cacao nibs (plus additional for topping)

- Toppings: more cacao nibs, goji berries, coconut, hemp seeds, sliced fresh strawberries

Instructions

1. Add banana, frozen strawberries, almond milk, ground flax, and cacao nibs to blender and pulse until creamy.

2. Transfer to bowl, add toppings and enjoy!

Mood Booster Smoothie

EQUIPMENT

• Blender

INGREDIENTS

• 1.5 cups Almond Milk or Oat Milk

• 1 Banana Ripe

• 1/3 cup Blackberries frozen

• 1/3 cup Raspberries frozen

• 1/3 cup Blueberries frozen

• 1 tbsp Honey adjust according to taste

• 1 tbsp Chia Seeds

• 1 tbsp Shredded Coconut to taste

INSTRUCTIONS

• Assemble your ingredients. Choose a ripe or overripe banana. Roughly chop banana for easier blending. Wash out your berries gently.

• Place all your ingredients into a clean blender, pouring the milk in, followed by the roughly chopped banana, blackberries and finally drizzle honey on the top.

• Blend away! Blend on medium for about 20 seconds. Check for any lumps. Blend for another 5 seconds on high speed to have a smooth lump-free smoothie full of bubbles.

• Your delicious, antioxidant packed smoothie is ready! Pour into a glass and top with coconut & fresh blueberries. Enjoy.

Mango Berry Double Layer Protein Smoothie

Category: Protein Smoothie

Servings: 1

Prep Time: 5 minutes

Ingredients

• Berry Layer (Bottom)

• ½ Cup Almond Milk

• ½ Cup Frozen Berries (Strawberries, Blueberries and Raspberries)

• 2 Scoops Greens + Reds Potent Immune Support

• ½ Cup Ice

• Mango Layer (Top)

• ½ Cup Almond Milk

• ½ Cup Fresh Mango

• ½ Cup Frozen Mango

• ½ Cup Ice

Directions

1. Add ingredients for bottom layer to Vitamix container in order listed.

2. Secure Lid, Blend on high, or smoothie setting until smooth.

3. Fill glass halfway.

4. Rinse Vitamix container.

5. Add ingredients for top layer to Vitamix container in order listed.

6. Secure Lid, Blend on high, or smoothie setting until smooth.

7. Fill the rest of the glass and enjoy!

CONCLUSION

Observational studies have shown that stroke risk-factors can be managed by improving nutritional intake. Most interventional studies have failed to achieve meaningful clinical outcomes. More research is needed to improve the quality of evidence, relating to the association of many nutrients, foods, and dietary patterns with stroke risk. To establish a causative role for specific nutrients, foods, and dietary patterns in the pathogenesis of stroke, adequately powered, large randomized trials are needed in which the patient population and intervention are carefully described and the outcomes not only, include all strokes but also, distinguish first-ever and recurrent stroke, and pathological, and etiological subtypes of stroke. To examine, the effects of interactions between different genetic and environmental factors, large genetic epidemiological studies that minimize bias, confounding, measurement errors, and random errors are needed.

Diets for stroke patients can vary depending on their exact needs. Often, it includes making changes to help avoid future strokes. This can involve eating foods that promote cardiovascular health, such as fruits, vegetables, whole grains, and lean proteins.

For people who have difficulty preparing food, eating, swallowing, or helping prevent weight loss, diet may also involve modifications that make these activities easier. For example, soft foods can be easier to eat while still giving a person the nutrients they need.

A person should contact a doctor or dietitian for advice on what to eat following a stroke, especially if they have other health conditions that have their own dietary requirements. Eat Healthier.

www.ingramcontent.com/pod-product-compliance
Lightning Source LLC
Chambersburg PA
CBHW061040250726
48653CB00001B/178